W9-CGU-343

D0123351

THE
ACTIVE
CAL RIE
DIET™

THE ACTIVE CALRIE DIET™

EAT MORE, **BURN MORE**, **LOSE MORE** WITH OUR
BREAKTHROUGH 4-WEEK PROGRAM

LESLIE BONCI, RD, with Selene Yeager and the Editors of **Prevention.**

RODALE

This book is intended as a reference volume only, not as a medical manual. The information given here is designed to help you make informed decisions about your health. It is not intended as a substitute for any treatment that may have been prescribed by your doctor. If you suspect that you have a medical problem, we urge you to seek competent medical help.

The information in this book is meant to supplement, not replace, proper exercise training. All forms of exercise pose some inherent risks. The editors and publisher advise readers to take full responsibility for their safety and know their limits. Before practicing the exercises in this book, be sure that your equipment is well-maintained, and do not take risks beyond your level of experience, aptitude, training, and fitness. The exercise and dietary programs in this book are not intended as a substitute for any exercise routine or dietary regimen that may have been prescribed by your doctor. As with all exercise and dietary programs, you should get your doctor's approval before beginning.

Mention of specific companies, organizations, or authorities in this book does not imply endorsement by the author or publisher, nor does mention of specific companies, organizations, or authorities imply that they endorse this book, its author, or the publisher.

Internet addresses and telephone numbers given in this book were accurate at the time it went to press.

To my husband, Fred; my sons, Gregory and Cary;
my parents, Annabelle and Jay; and my brother, Louis

And to our fabulous participants: Natalie Wingard; Carol Steig;
Camilla Monti; Irwin Shapiro; Bill Ankrom; Kathleen Schmidt;
Jeannette Johnson; Patty Speicher; Carol Semple Thompson;
Cherry Semple White; Karen Quinn; Jackie Detty; Wendy Keirn;
Deborah Griffin; Suzanne Coglio; Melissa Shilling; and Kim Wagner.
Your willingness, enthusiasm, and hard work turned an idea
into a reality. THANK YOU!
—Leslie

For my family. Without your support,
none of this would have been possible.
—Selene

Contents

Acknowledgments

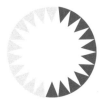

Words cannot begin to describe how grateful I am to Selene, an accomplished writer, athlete par excellence, and coconspirator.

Thank you, Andrea, editor extraordinaire, and Marielle, who kept us accountable and everything flowing like clockwork.

To Jennifer, for providing the savor and flavor to the plate, bowl, and plan!

To Fred, my voice of reason, whose patience, encouragement, and support through the writing process make me forever grateful.

To my patients, who have enlightened my life and fine-tuned my professional skills.

To my colleagues, for your insight, suggestions, and enthusiasm.

To my employer, Dr. Freddie Fu, whose unwavering support and vision compel me to strive.

And a heartfelt thanks to our test panel participants. We couldn't have done it without you. You learned how to activate, initiate, and collaborate. BRAVO!

—*Leslie*

This book was truly a team effort, and I'd like to thank the tremendous people who made it happen: Leslie Bonci, a perfect project partner; Jennifer Iserloh, for delicious, creative recipe planning; Andrea Au Levitt, for her undying patience and positivity; Marielle Messing, for taking the reins and running; Joanna Williams and Carol Angstadt, for the gorgeous design; Susan Eugster and Mitch Mandel, for the fabulous photos; and all the test panelists who brought the Active Calorie Diet to life.   —*Selene*

Introduction

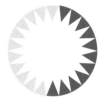

Calories:

It's Not about Counting Them; It's about Making Them Count

I've been a nutritionist for 2 decades. I work with professional and recreational athletes of all shapes and sizes. I work with office workers. I work with stay-at-home moms. I work with kids and seniors. I guess you could say I've seen it all. But I'll tell you what—over all the years and all the thousands of clients, some things never change. Dieting is one of them.

Without fail, when someone walks through my door, I know what I'm going to hear: "I'm ready to make sweeping changes. Just tell me what I can't eat." It's all about how low can you go, deprivation, and punishment. People have this misguided notion that food is bad. That eating is somehow an evil activity to be avoided with all the will-power one can muster. That they're weak if they give in to the temptations of the table. They villainize food, especially the foods they like. Everyone wants a diet—the more spartan the better. Much to their great disappointment, I never give it to them. Why? Because for one, I don't believe in deprivation; and frankly, I know it doesn't work.

Or, I should say, it doesn't work over the long term. Anyone, but anyone, can lose lots of weight by following a diet for a few months. She may be miserable the whole time, but she can bite the bullet and do it. But then what happens? She can't wait to stop. And when she finally does, all those pounds and then some come piling back on. I have plenty of clients who have lost 100 pounds by losing and gaining the same 20 over and over again. Maybe you relate. Don't feel bad. It's not your fault. Diets simply do not work, because they leave you feeling hungry, grumpy, and unsatisfied.

What does work? Satiety (pronounced "sat-EYE-ity"). It's nutritionist-speak for feeling pleasantly full. Think about it. When are you most happy after eating? When the meal you've just eaten has left you satisfied but not stuffed. When you feel full and energetic. You don't get that from a deprivation diet. You get headachy, low-energy, cranky spells followed by out-of-control binges that make you feel miserable and defeated and also encourage your body to store fat and increase your weight. You know what else you don't get from those diets? A healthy metabolism. Everyone wants to "spark," "rev," and "ramp up" their metabolism. But then they skip breakfast and sometimes lunch and otherwise starve themselves, which dims those calorie-burning furnaces to a flicker.

The Active Calorie plan is not about what you need to take out of your diet; it's about what you need to put into it. It's more about what to add than what to take away. It's firmly grounded in science. It's tested on real women and men just like you. And it works. In just 4 weeks, five of the test-panel volunteers dropped a full size or more. But the weight loss alone is not what tells me that it really works. As we were interviewing the participants, they all said the same things:

"I never felt deprived."

"I'm definitely going to continue eating this way. My whole family loves it."

"I'm not on a diet. I just finally know how to eat better."

"It's not rigid at all. I just follow the Active Calorie Plate guidelines, and I can eat right anywhere."

"I'm going to do this forever!"

That's how I know this plan delivers without deprivation.

You Are as You Eat

Before we even talk food, the first thing I want you to add to your diet is time. Listen, I know you're busy. These days, there are precious few people who can say they aren't crazy busy, booked solid. Yet we find time for what is important to us. Nielsen data show that we watch 4 hours and 35 minutes of TV a day. We surf the Net for hours catching up on Facebook, Twitter, and other social media sites. I'm not asking you to unplug your life. But I am asking you to spend a little more time tuning in to your relationship with the food that nourishes you. That includes spending just a little more time buying your food as well as preparing and eating it. We're not transporting you back to the 1950s or asking you to slave for hours over a hot stove. Just do a little more than roll down the car window and order a No. 3 combo meal with a soda.

For decades we've been trying to decipher the secret of the enviably thin women in France and other European countries, who seemingly stay effortlessly thin despite their penchant for croissants, butter, cream sauces, and other "fattening" foods. Reams of books and articles have been written claiming that it's the red wine or the olive oil that keeps them slender. But honestly, it's their approach to food, from start to finish. For one, they really think about their food. They stop at the market several times a week, if not every day, to pick up fresh vegetables, fruits, bread, and meat. They take time to prepare simple yet nourishing meals. And most important, they sit down at a table—usually with family and/or friends—and they take time to really eat. They don't grab, gulp, and go the way we do far too often in this country, barely remembering what or where we've eaten 10 minutes after we've wiped the crumbs from our laps. They enjoy their food. They put their forks down between bites to carry on a conversation and savor the flavors of the dish. They eat more slowly. They chew thoroughly. And ultimately they eat less.

That's their great secret. And guess what? When they start adopting a drive-thru eating lifestyle, they get fat, too. We're starting to see this in places across the globe—even China, where obesity has been long unheard of—when real meals are replaced by fast food. It's time to turn that tide around.

Stop Counting Calories

It always surprises me that so many people are willing to pour hours of energy into counting calories but not nearly as much into where those calories are coming from. They'll drink unsatisfying shakes, eat microscopic meal bars, and subsist on cabbage soup so long as they nail a certain calorie quota that they believe will help them lose weight fast. That works on paper. But your body isn't made of paper. It's made of flesh and blood and billions of cells that need nourishment to function optimally, which is the real ticket to weight loss. That's why the Active Calorie Diet isn't about counting calories; it's about making them count.

Contrary to what you've been led to believe, not all calories are created equal. How your body processes, burns, and stores them depends on where they come from. Believe it or not, studies have found that eating fat is necessary for burning fat. That's right. Eat the right kinds of fat, and your body burns more of the calories you eat. (Ever wonder why the low-fat craze made us all fatter? This is part of the reason.) Ditto for protein. Textbooks tell us that protein contains 4 calories per gram. Now we know that's not entirely true. Research shows that protein boosts your metabolism so much (because digesting and processing it is a lot of work) that its calorie count should be dropped 20 percent so that it's actually closer to 3 calories per gram. Other metabolism starters—which I call Active Calories—include high-fiber foods like beans, nuts, and veggies, all of which require so much work from your body to process that you burn more calories all day after eating them than you would by eating a typical highly refined diet, which leaves your body with little to do other than store fat.

The Active Calorie Diet takes advantage of these high-energy foods by adding more of them to your diet. Then we fan the flames even further by tossing in foods and drinks and spices—such as chile peppers, coffee, tea, cinnamon, and ginger—that turn up your metabolism to high. You'll find a complete list in Chapter 5, along with almost 80 complete recipes that pull it all together in Chapter 7.

On the flip side, you can bring your metabolism to a grinding halt by consuming too many of what I call Couch Potato Calories (you'll find a whole chapter on these starting on page 45), such as highly refined, starchy foods; juices; and artificial fats and sweeteners. As you'll see in Chapter 4, research shows that even if you don't overeat these foods, you may still gain weight (or at least not lose any) because they slow your metabolism and are so easily digested that in the end, you absorb and store more of the calories you eat. You heard that right. You can eat the same number of Active Calories and Couch Potato Calories but lose weight from the former and gain it from the latter, simply because of what happens to those calories once they enter your body.

By changing your plate to add more Active Calories, you will stimulate your body to burn more energy, blunt your appetite to slow down the flow of calories, fire up your fat-burning engines, and more. As a bonus, Active Calories not only help you lose weight but also help you be more active, so you burn fat and firm up even faster.

Eat—Then Get Off Your Seat

The Active Calorie Diet is not an exercise book. But you will find a chapter that includes strength training, stretching, and cardio because those are essential weight loss and weight maintenance tools. More important, I want you to be more active in your everyday life (which you automatically will be in the kitchen if you follow the food-prepping recommendations).

Here's the deal. Thanks to modern conveniences such as Internet shopping, online banking, e-mailing, texting, and computer- and phone-driven working and even socializing, we now burn up to 1,000 fewer calories than we did just 30 years ago. If you're like the average laptop-loving, cell phone–worshipping, hardworking man or woman in the electronic age, you likely spend a stunning 56 hours a week planted like a begonia—staring at your computer screen, slumped behind the steering wheel, tapping your iPhone, or collapsed in a heap in front of your high-def TV. And it's killing you. Literally. All this downtime is so unhealthy that it's given birth to a new realm of medical study—inactivity physiology, which explores the ramifications of our increasingly sedentary lives—and a deadly new epidemic: sitting disease. And it's not something that can be undone by 30 minutes on the treadmill 4 or 5 days a week.

In one study of 168 men and women, researchers from the University of Queensland in Australia found that regardless of how much (or how little) moderate to vigorous exercise the volunteers did, those who took more breaks from sitting had slimmer waists, lower BMIs, and healthier blood-fat and blood-sugar levels than those who sat the most.[1] (Your BMI, or body mass index, gives a picture of your total body fat in proportion to your overall height and weight and is a more accurate indicator of healthy weight than pounds alone.) In an extensive lifestyle study of 17,000 men and women, Canadian researchers drew an even more succinct conclusion: The longer you spend sitting, the more likely you are to die an early death.[2] You're also more likely to be overweight . . . and unhappy.

That's why the Active Calorie Diet puts such a high premium on everyday activity. Chopping vegetables, grating cheese, strolling the supermarket aisles for just the right spices, and becoming a truly active participant in your eating burns serious calories! Not each incidental move in and of itself, of course. But collectively, these small movements make up the bulk of your energy expenditure and can be the difference between being lean and being overweight. I recommend taking many minibreaks throughout the day to get off your seat. You'll find specific strategies in Chapter 9.

Awareness Is Everything

Old habits die hard—especially old, mindless habits like munching your way through a bag of chips while watching the Cowboys play the Colts or downing one or two doughnuts during your Monday-morning meeting at work, simply because they're there. The problem with these eating episodes is that, one, they're nearly always in the form of Couch Potato Calories; and two, we barely register them, so over the course of a day, we eat far more than we intend. Don't feel bad about it. We all have nearly unconscious food triggers—events, places, even friends and family—that trip a switch in us that sends us to the chips and dip. That's why I ask you to keep a food journal for the 4 weeks of the Active Calorie Diet.

Journaling is not just a worthwhile activity in its own right; writing down what you eat, why you're eating, how full you are, and how it makes you feel will help you pinpoint and, if necessary, avoid or adapt to these food triggers. One of my clients never realized what a huge food trigger her mother was until she started writing down everything she ate while inside the walls of her childhood home. The answer wasn't to avoid her mother, a loving Italian woman who believed in feeding—really feeding—her children, but to figure out a way she could take her mother's gifts without giving up on the Active Calorie life.

The solution was surprisingly simple. She didn't have to eat every morsel during her visit. She could take some of the food with her. She ate more slowly and deliberately while she was there, so her mother never saw an empty plate. Then, when her mother offered more food, she said, "Could I get it to go? I'd love to have more of this for later." As you can imagine, her mother was more than happy to oblige! Meanwhile, just being aware that she was eating was enough to make her eat less. "I stopped reading while I was eating," she told me. "I'd start a meal and look down, and it would be gone. I wouldn't even remember eating it!"

Along the same lines, I'm also asking you to journal your physical activity for these 4 weeks. Again, the goal isn't to torture you by making you write down all the minutiae of your day. The goal is awareness. I want you to be aware of the sedentary spots in your routine. I want you to find places where you can "activate" your day by getting up and moving around. It can be as easy as standing up when you check and respond to e-mail. Writing down your daily activities raises your awareness and helps make your new Active Calorie life habits more permanent.

Make It Happen

I wrote this book because I know that people need change they can live with. Short-term diets are just that: short term. You lose the weight; you stop the diet; you put the weight back on. Many people live their whole lives that way. I'd like to give you a better, sustainable option that you can implement for the rest of your life to stay trim and healthy rather than yo-yoing up and down on the scale indefinitely.

I wrote this book because I know people are terribly confused about calories. There's so much information and misinformation. Let's face it: Even the USDA's Food Pyramid isn't much help. Nobody knows what a serving is or what they're actually supposed to eat from meal to meal. Easily 80 percent of the members of the volunteer test panel admitted to being confused about what foods (and how much food) they should really eat. The Active Calorie Plate, which you'll learn more about in Chapters 1 and 5, removes the guesswork and makes it crystal clear where your (active) calories should be coming from during breakfast, lunch, dinner, and snacks.

I wrote this book because I know this method works. In fact, it changes lives. But don't just take my word for it. Here's what Camilla Monti, 60, who lost 9 pounds and 2½ inches off her waist in 4 weeks, had to say of her experience: "I have a PhD in dieting. I've been dieting for decades. I've never been able to lose 10 pounds in a year, let alone a few weeks! My boyfriend has seen it all, and he's surprised I've really stuck with it this time. But it's easy to do. It's working. And I'm not stopping!"

Now it's your turn. Flip the pages and let your Active Calorie life begin.

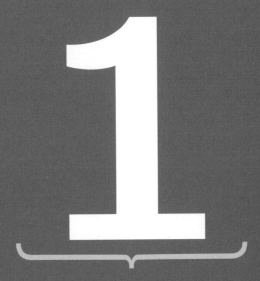

1

Eat More:
What Is an Active Calorie?

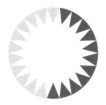

Calories. If you're like most women (or men) trying to lose weight, calories are a big part of your life. You count them. You save them. You splurge on them. You do your darndest to burn as many of them as you can. But is it working? If you're like 67 percent of women who are perennially (and not so successfully) trying to lose weight and keep it off, the answer is no. Why? Because until now, what you've been told about calories isn't entirely true.

For years we have been told that when it comes to weight loss, a calorie is a calorie (is a calorie). It doesn't matter if you eat 500 calories' worth of celery or 500 buried beneath the crispy crust of a crème brûlée—your body will burn and/or store them equally. I'm here to tell you that this is simply not true. Researchers have uncovered new science that shows that when it comes to weight loss, calories are anything but equal. That's why counting calories can be such a colossal waste of time. It doesn't work, because what we've been taught is incorrect.

That's right. A *New Scientist* feature aptly titled "The Calorie Delusion" explains it simply: Calorie counts are based on the numbers generated by a machine. But human bodies are not machines. We do not incinerate calories. We digest them. From chewing to swallowing to chemical breakdown and processing, how those calories act within our bodies varies widely from food to food. One simple but very important factor is how much work the body must do to break down and process each bite. I, along with many other researchers around the globe, believe that this one factor alone may be responsible for a large portion of our runaway-obesity crisis.

The Calorie Equation

The calorie concept that so many of us live and diet by is grounded in a system developed back in the 19th century by American chemist Wilbur Olin Atwater. To determine how what we eat gives us energy, Atwater burned small samples of various foods in controlled conditions and measured the amount of energy released in the form of heat. Then he calculated the amount of energy that would be lost in undigested food parts (such as fiber) as well as in our waste products. The calorie counts he arrived at—and they are ballparks, not absolutes—have stood as gospel ever since.

Problem is, over the past 150 years, a lot has changed about how—and what—we eat. Before microwaves, white bread, and fast food, people ate mostly whole foods that they bought at the market or grew in their own backyards. When you eat foods that are close to their natural state—like fruits, vegetables, whole grains, and lean cuts of meat—your body has to work to eat them. You need to work to chew them. You need to work to digest them. They create what scientists call a thermic response, which means that you burn calories just by processing them. Because whole foods are more difficult to digest and have more matter that is indigestible, your body doesn't necessarily absorb all the calories from those foods, either. Not only does the process consume energy, but a high percentage of the food just passes through. It's not so easy to get all the calories out of beans, broccoli, or brown rice. These are Active Calories.

In contrast, take a look at the french fries, bagels, pastries, pasta, chicken nuggets, burgers, pizza, and other processed foods that we love so much for their convenience. That fast-food chicken sandwich has gone through so much pulverization, you barely have to chew. The whole digestive process is being bypassed from the beginning, and we're losing the ability to burn calories as we would naturally. In short, it's easy for our bodies to take in all the calories from an overcooked potato, a ground-up burger, a glass of juice, or a Boston cream doughnut. These are what I call Couch Potato Calories.

Think such small changes in our food supply couldn't possibly make such a big impact on our collective belly size? Think again. In a study published in the *American Journal of Clinical Nutrition*, Japanese researchers surveyed 450 female students about their eating habits and then classified the food they ate according to how difficult it was to chew. Across the board, those who ate the foods that required the most work had significantly slimmer waistlines than those who ate the softest, easiest-to-eat foods.[1]

Animal studies are equally striking. In another study out of Japan, researchers fed one group of rats their usual hard food pellets and served a similar group of rats pellets that had the same nutritional and calorie content but had been softened so that they were easier to chew. After just 5½ months, the rats that dined on the softened food had actually gained enough weight to be classified as obese and had higher levels of deep, dangerous belly fat, while the rats eating their normal chow had no such changes.[2] Simply changing the texture of food is enough to trick your body into storing more belly-bloating fat. Many of the Active Calorie test panelists were shocked at how full they felt and for how long on the Active Calorie Diet. "I could polish off an entire box of Oreos or a big bag of chips and still be hungry, but I couldn't even finish some of the breakfasts on this diet," one of the panelists told me.

That's just the beginning. As you'll soon discover, there's more to Active Calories than texture. During my 20-plus years overhauling my clients' diets, I've discovered a gold mine of Active Calories—all supported by solid scientific evidence, as well as many happy clients and pounds lost. In the Active Calorie Diet, I target four specific types of

Active Calories—chewy, hearty, energizing, and warming (CHEW for short)—that will help you lose weight simply by eating! That's right. You'll learn about dozens of foods that will not only stimulate your body to burn more energy but also blunt your appetite to slow down the flow of calories.

Your meals will elevate your resting energy expenditure (that's your metabolism), so your fat-burning engines will be set on high all day long. What you eat will even boost the number of calories you burn when you work out. One British study published in the *Journal of Nutrition* found that when women ate a breakfast rich in fiber-rich "hearty" Active Calories, they burned twice as much fat during a 60-minute walk later that morning than when they started the day with Couch Potato Calories.[3] Why is that? Because Couch Potato Calories sail from your belly to your bloodstream in the blink of an eye, spiking your blood sugar, which your body then burns when you walk or exercise. Hearty calories are digested more slowly, so your body has to pull energy from your fat stores as well.

What else will Active Calories do for you? How about lower your risk of heart disease, diabetes, and even some types of cancer? How? By making your body work the way it was meant to work. When your digestive system is fully engaged with the proper flow of food, your blood sugar remains level and controlled; you're less likely to overeat; and, as mentioned earlier, you increase your body's ability to burn fat—especially the deep abdominal fat that smothers your heart and other internal organs, driving up your blood pressure as well as your triglyceride and cholesterol levels.

Finally, by filling up on Active Calories, you're effectively cutting the number of calories your body will store because you're burning more and absorbing fewer than you would if you ate the same number of Couch Potato Calories. Protein-rich foods make your body work so hard to digest them that you burn about 20 percent of the calories from those foods just by processing them. Warming foods like hot peppers can raise your metabolic rate 5 percent. As you'll soon see, even certain carbs can crank up your calorie burn.

But don't just take my—or other scientists'—word for it. Take it from Suzanne Coglio, 48, who lost 12 pounds in just 1 month of eating a diet chock-full of Active Calories. "I love that this diet is grounded in real food. We weren't forced to eat bland foods like cottage cheese or to be so restricted that there's nothing you really want to eat," she says. "There are so many foods and combinations of foods in this plan that I would never have thought to try. It's been terrific. Now, instead of dreading eating, like I do on so many diets, I look forward to it. I've been very surprised by just how good good-for-you foods could be! And they're all real, flexible food choices you can live with. I love it."

The best part: Not only is the food delicious, easy to prepare, and good for you, but it will also make you feel good. You'll have more, longer-lasting energy and fewer blood-sugar spikes and crashes. In addition, the meals you eat will leave you happy, full, and satisfied instead of rummaging through the kitchen cabinets 30 minutes later.

Eat More!

Active Calories do you no good unless you eat them. That's right: You must eat to lose weight. That will surely come as a surprise to so many women (and men) who have been taught that calories—all calories—are the enemy to be avoided at any cost. Admit it: You've probably skipped meals in hopes of shedding pounds. Lots of people have. A survey presented at the 2008 International Conference on Eating Disorders in Seattle reported that 37 percent of women regularly skip meals to lose weight, more than a quarter cut out entire food groups, and 16 percent have winnowed their calories down to 1,000 a day or fewer.[4] Those are all huge mistakes. Cutting calories, especially Active Calories, can be the worst thing for your energy-burning metabolism and, therefore, weight loss.

The classic calorie equations tell us that each pound is worth 3,500 calories. For healthy, sustainable weight loss—about a pound a week—that means cutting your usual intake by 500 calories a day. That's the equivalent of two regular sodas and half a bagel. Some men

(continued on page 8)

{ carol semple thompson }

Feeding an Active Life

AGE: 61
POUNDS LOST
14
INCHES LOST:
7¾ including 4 inches off her waist

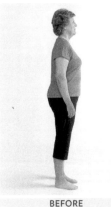

BEFORE

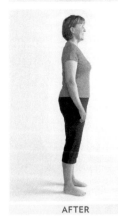

AFTER

AN ACTIVE LIFE and the Active Calorie Diet go together like sun and surf—they're both pleasant on their own, but they're twice as nice together. Nobody on the test panel exemplified that quite as perfectly as Carol Semple Thompson, who, as a professional golfer, understands all too well how what you eat can affect how you play. When Carol came to us, she was simply tired of feeling so tired. She traveled and ate out a lot as part of her job. She just wanted to get a sense of what her plate should look like so she could shed some stubborn pounds and have more energy. Boy, did she ever.

"There's so much food when you're on the road. It's hard to know what the best options are. I didn't think I ate too poorly, but the pounds have been creeping on, and my energy has been waning," she told me during our initial meeting. "I can't follow a diet to the letter. And I need a plan that allows for some flexibility, because I'm on the road with only so many food choices available to me. I need a diet that I can adjust to my lifestyle." Carol found it in the Active Calorie Diet, which she did with her sister Cherry (see page 50). The single element she found most useful: the Active Calorie Plate (see Chapter 5).

"I have gotten such a great benefit from just looking at that plate and making sure that mine looks like that, with the right amount of protein and vegetables. That's been huge for me," says Carol, who dropped 14 pounds in a month without ever feeling that she was really dieting.

It also helped her figure out portion control, a concept that had eluded her, especially when she was eating out. "Now I make sure I have the right elements in my meal, and I simply don't eat everything that's served to me. And that's okay," she says. "The hardest part is when we have to sit for a long dinner and they keep bringing out more and more bread. That's a little challenging. But it's not that big a deal. If the dessert is really good, I'll have a little of that. In the end I feel so much better, it's worth it." Carol has also achieved a new level of mindfulness that helps her eat better in every situation. "I used to eat when I was bored or just as something to do," she told me. Now she thinks ahead to situations in which she might be tempted into mindless munching. "Now I'll occupy myself with something besides a bag of snacks when I'm in the car for long trips to the next tournament. A little fruit and audiobooks keep me great company," she says with a satisfied smile. "This is something I can definitely keep doing."

and women, eager for faster results, slice their calorie consumption even more deeply. But your body isn't so easily starved into submission. I've seen clients subsisting on a few hundred calories' worth of weight loss shakes every day who come in completely frustrated and discouraged because the scale simply won't budge. Why? Because they're eating so little, their metabolism is set on snooze.

Your body has a baseline metabolic rate—the minimum amount of energy (calories) that it needs to carry out its basic housekeeping functions, such as breathing, thinking, circulating blood, and digesting food. If you cut your calories below that point, your body will protect you by slowing down your metabolism, which of course means fewer calories burned and pounds lost. Generally speaking, ladies, your baseline metabolic rate is your goal weight times 10. (Guys, for you, it's your goal weight times 11.) So if you want to be 130 pounds, it's 1,300 calories. Then add another 200 for your daily activity (housework, walking around at work, and general milling about). In my practice (and in much of the literature), I have found that the minimum number of calories you should consume for weight loss is 1,500 for "reasonably" active women (meaning you get out and walk or otherwise do a little physical activity for 20 to 30 minutes a few times a week) and 1,800 for reasonably active men. Those are the figures I use for the Active Calorie menus, and it's an amount that most of you will find is filling and fulfilling while still being low enough to peel off pounds and keep them off. If you are completely sedentary, I recommend getting up and getting active (you'll find many ways in this book!) to burn a couple hundred calories a day rather than slicing your intake any further. It's more effective for firing up your fat-burning metabolism and far better for your general health.

Eat Regularly

The last piece in the new calorie equation isn't just what you eat and how much but when. I'll start with the most essential: Don't skip meals—ever—especially breakfast. Your body needs calories at regular intervals to keep your metabolism humming along. The number one error of dieters nationwide is missing the most important meal of all: breakfast.

When you skip breakfast—and/or lunch, for that matter (yes, I've had clients who "righteously" brag about being able to skip both)—you not only start your day with your metabolism fully suppressed but also set yourself up for overeating later in the day, when your brain cells scream "Enough!" and send you to the refrigerator to stuff down everything in sight. A study published in the *British Journal of Nutrition* found that this commonly practiced "gorging pattern" of food intake prompts your body to pack on weight and increases fat formation, likely because your body thinks that food is scarce, so it wants to store every morsel you devour when you finally feed it.[5]

Regular eating reverses that metabolism-dimming process. Eating breakfast in particular throws it into high gear. A morning meal raises your metabolism and prevents weight gain. Front-loading your day with adequate calories is also an easy way to lose weight because you'll be less hungry as the day goes on and thus less likely to succumb to the calls of the vending machine or those leftover cookies hanging out in the office pantry. In one study published in the *American Journal of Epidemiology*, men and women who ate 22 to 55 percent of their daily calories at breakfast gained an average of only 1.7 pounds over 4 years, compared with about 3 pounds gained among their peers who ate zero to 11 percent of their calories in the morning.[6] Another study published in the same journal reported that people who regularly skip breakfast were $4\frac{1}{2}$ times more likely to be overweight or obese than those who ate a morning meal.[7] You'll also have more energy to prepare healthful meals, exercise (and burn calories), and otherwise up your activity level—not to mention, you'll be happier and more focused on your tasks for the day.

Though I am a fan of eating regularly, I'm no fan of a trend that started about a decade ago that I would like to see end: snacking all day under the guise of "minimeals." This so-called grazing is more suitable for farm animals than for human beings. The original intent of eating every 2 to 3 hours was to keep your blood-sugar levels stable so you never got too hungry. But the problem is that now everyone is eating all the time and has forgotten the virtues of feeling hunger. Grazing also makes it extremely easy to overeat.

Theoretically, if you're eating six minimeals a day, each should contain no more than 250 to 300 calories. That's the amount in a bowl of cereal and a small glass of orange juice. Maybe you limit yourself to so few calories at breakfast (when you should actually be eating more) or for a snack, but when is the last time you had a 250-calorie dinner? Or even lunch? Instead, people are eating three regular meals plus three (at least) snacks. If you never feel hungry (and then satisfied after eating), how will you know how much you actually do—or don't—need to eat? Grazing also leads to mindless eating. People are noshing on string cheese, crackers, granola, and lots and lots of empty calories for all sorts of reasons that have nothing to do with being hungry. You'll never lose weight that way.

The Active Calorie Diet celebrates food. It celebrates eating full, satisfying meals in reasonable increments. It asks that you pay attention to your food choices and how they make you feel. It also lets you enjoy feeling the relative fullness that comes with eating a bigger meal. I'm not antisnack. There's room for a snack in your day, but just one well-timed snack to hold you over between meals. In most cases, this snack works best in the midafternoon, especially if you don't tend to eat dinner until closer to 7:00 p.m. Like your meals, your snacks should be a balanced mix of Active Calories, including foods high in chewy, hearty, energizing, and/or warming calories.

Eat Real Food

So now that I've just told you all about calories and how many you need and don't need, I'm going to tell you not to get caught up in trying to count them obsessively. Counting calories takes the joy out of eating and, in my experience, usually ends up being a futile venture unless you're willing to measure and weigh every morsel. Instead, fill your plate with Active Calories from real, whole, natural foods.

The closer foods are to their natural state, the more fiber and water they have, which means they get digested slowly, leave you feeling satisfied with less, and provide longer-lasting energy. By changing the composition of your plate, you can lose weight without worrying about counting calories, wrangling with hunger pangs and crankiness, or feeling as if you're running on fumes. You'll find a complete discussion of this topic in Chapter 5. But here's what Active Calorie eating looks like at a glance.

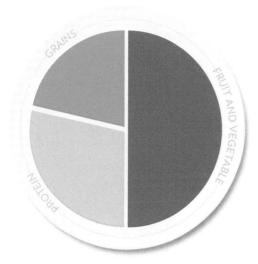

■ Fruit/Vegetable ▨ Protein ■ Grains

A little more than a quarter of the plate should be chewy Active Calories from protein such as lean meat, skinless poultry, fish, soy foods, eggs, or low-fat dairy. This is about a palm-size amount of food, or about 4 ounces of cooked-weight food.

About half of the plate should be chewy and hearty Active Calories from fresh fruits and vegetables. This should be about two fist-size servings of fruits and/or vegetables.

A little less than a quarter of the plate should be hearty Active Calories from whole grain carbs such as brown rice, whole wheat pasta, potatoes, or tortillas (preferably whole wheat). A serving of these should be about the size of your fist, or 1 cup.

To help you get the hang of it, I've included 78 meals, desserts, and snacks in Chapter 7 and a 4-week meal plan in Appendix B, which automatically give you the appropriate number of calories. Follow the plan for 1 full month, paying attention to the size of the portions and the composition of your meals. After these few weeks, you'll learn to put together healthy, properly portioned Active Calorie meals on your own.

The Active Calorie Diet encourages you to cook more and take a more active role in your meal planning and preparation. But I don't live in a bubble. I know that life is crazy busy, and eating out and grabbing takeout is sometimes a must. That's why, in Chapter 8, I've included dozens of samples of perfect Active Calorie fast-food choices and Active Calorie meals that you'll find at popular fast-casual restaurants.

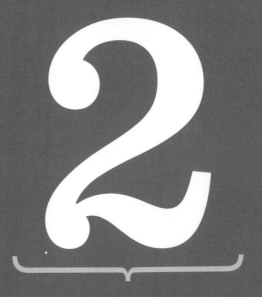

Burn More:
The Thermic Effect of Food

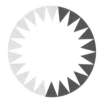

Too many people view eating as a guilty pleasure rather than a pleasurable way to feed their bodies and fuel themselves for an active life. Does "guilty pleasure" describe your relationship with food? Do you think in terms of everything you "shouldn't" eat instead of all the great foods you can and should consume? Do you feel guilty after eating? If you answered yes to any of these questions, you're far from alone, and it's time for a change. It's time to think of eating—yes, eating, not depriving yourself of food—as a means to attaining and maintaining a lean, active body. That is the foundation of the Active Calorie plan: Eat food to lose weight.

The Active Calorie approach to eating is far more effective than shakes, juice fasts, deprivation, and spartan diets that eliminate entire food groups, because it works the way your body is intended to work: by eating and digesting real, whole foods. Each forkful you eat boosts your metabolism by triggering the release of hormones and enzymes and making your body work to break down food and turn it into energy. It's something that most of us never consider: Eating requires energy—lots of energy, if you eat the right foods. Unfortunately, most of us have been unknowingly eating the wrong ones. Even foods we think are healthful, like commercial juices and "whole grain" breads, have often been so processed that we barely have to chew, let alone digest, them. This not only robs us of hours of elevated calorie burn but also increases the number of calories we stash away as fat.

So how do we identify the right foods that contain the Active Calories that require our bodies to burn more energy? We look at what's called the thermic effect of food, the calorie-burn bump we get from eating and digesting any given type of food. In the past, this phenomenon was known as the "specific dynamic action" of food, which, though more of a mouthful, tells a better story. I've studied weight management and digestive health for the better part of 20 years. I assure you, the entire process of picking, preparing, chewing, swallowing, digesting, and processing calories can be a series of extremely dynamic actions that are very specific to the foods you eat.

Chews to Lose

Digestion starts before you take your first bite. Seeing and smelling and anticipating food unleashes a cascade of digestive messenger molecules—such as cholecystokinin, somatostatin, and neurotensin—that prep your digestive tract for the food to come. Just gazing at and soaking in the aroma of that grilled seafood salad is enough to increase production of these messengers by more than 50 percent.

The moment you put that first morsel in your mouth, the mechanics begin. At the most basic level, chewing food mechanically breaks down the large chunks into small bits that are easier to swallow. Foods that take more work to chew—such as nuts, a piece of lean meat, or even chewy whole grain rice—obviously use more mouth energy than a fluffy, cream-filled Twinkie does. They also put your entire digestive system into motion earlier. When you stimulate your taste receptors by chewing your food in a leisurely fashion, they stimulate your stomach lining to increase production of hydrochloric acid in order to break down the food coming its way and also send the message to your small intestines to ramp up their army of digestive enzymes and get ready for the job at hand.

As you chew on that strip of beef jerky, your body helps break it down by sending in more saliva. This food lubrication contains essential chemicals that help dissolve the bonds in the food to make the energy and nutrients easier to pull out and process. Chewing and the saliva it generates also help relax your pylorus, a muscle at the lower end of your stomach that shuttles food into your small intestine, leading the way for smooth, healthy digestion. The more you chew, the more signals your body sends out, readying the rest of your digestive tract for the food that is on the way.

Just the act of chewing—working your mandibles more—can increase your calorie burn by about 10 percent. In a study by Mayo Clinic researchers, volunteers who chewed gum (more on that in Chapter 3) for 12 minutes at 100 chews per hour increased their calorie burn by 11 calories—nearly 1 calorie per chew![1] Imagine how many more calories you could burn each and every day for the rest of your life simply by sitting down to really chew your food. That's what Active Calorie eating is about!

Burn after Eating

After chewing and partially digesting your food, you swallow it through your esophagus, sending it into the rest of your digestive factory, where your body sets about completely breaking down, absorbing, and storing the nutritious elements and ultimately eliminating the waste from each and every bite. It's a big job that starts as soon as you swallow your first mouthful and peaks about 2 to 3 hours after you've pushed away from the table. Exactly how much work (that is, calorie burn) does all that entail? Depends on what you've eaten (hint: Active Calories burn the most). This posteating after-burn can range anywhere from a measly flicker of a flame at 2 to 3 percent to a towering inferno of 25 to 30 percent. Here's how what you eat stacks up.

Protein: Thermic Effect, 25 to 30 Percent

When you follow the Active Calorie Diet, you'll be eating protein at every single meal and snack, for good reason: It is an essential ingredient for losing weight and keeping it off. Protein is a potent calorie burner because it's such a power player in nearly every bodily function. You likely know that you need protein to build strong, lean muscle, but you may not realize how this complex macronutrient weaves itself into nearly every fiber of your body. Far beyond just building shapely biceps, protein is an essential component of your hair, skin, hormones, enzymes—essentially, every cell. It's a major player in regulating immunity, sleep, digestion, and even ovulation. Protein builds bone; without it, you can eat all the calcium and vitamin D in the world but won't be able to absorb it and use it to create healthy bone mass. Protein also builds, repairs, and preserves metabolism-revving lean muscle tissue as you exercise and lose weight. In one study, dieters who followed the standard protein recommendations (10 to 15 percent of their calories) while shedding pounds lost nearly double the amount of lean muscle tissue (6.2 pounds), compared with those who boosted their protein intake to 30 percent of their calories while they lost weight.[2]

All of those physical processes take a lot of energy—and protein, which most of us simply don't get enough of. Upping your intake will not only speed your weight loss but also keep you healthier, according to recent research. A Johns Hopkins University study found that a diet in which about 25 percent of the calories—about 60 percent more than the recommended 10 to 15 percent—came from lean-protein sources reduced blood pressure, LDL-cholesterol levels, and triglycerides better than a traditional higher-carb diet did.[3] Other research finds that diets with higher levels of protein can help prevent obesity, osteoporosis, and diabetes. Tilting your diet in favor of protein may even help you live longer. The OmniHeart (Optimal Macronutrient Intake Trial to Prevent Heart Disease) study reported that men and women who switched from a diet that was 58 percent carbs and 15 percent protein to one that was

48 percent carbs and 25 percent protein lowered their 10-year risk of heart disease by nearly 30 percent.[4]

High-protein foods really are your best ally in the Active Calorie Diet. They take more work to chew and longer to leave your stomach, so you take more time eating (and have more time to register that you're full). They also slow down the release of carbs and fat into your bloodstream. You feel full sooner and stay satisfied longer. The cumulative effect can help you lose nearly a pound a week without doing anything else. In one study, dieters who increased their protein intake to 30 percent of their diets ate nearly 450 fewer calories a day and lost about 11 pounds over the 12-week study without trying.[5] I especially like to start the day with plenty of protein. One study in the International Journal of Obesity reported that men and women dieters who cracked two eggs for breakfast lost 65 percent more weight and had a 34 percent greater reduction in their waistlines than those who ate a bagel for their morning meal.[6] "I never ate protein in the morning before," says Debe Griffin, who lost nearly 10 pounds on the plan. "I can't believe how much fuller I feel."

Though all protein falls under the Active Calorie umbrella, some sources are superior to others. Protein is made up of 20 building blocks called amino acids. Of these, your body makes 11, which are called nonessential amino acids. The other nine, known as essential amino acids, you need to get from food. If you're looking for one-stop sources of complete protein, look no further than animal products. All animal products—including red meat, poultry, eggs, dairy, and fish—are complete proteins, meaning they contain all nine essential amino acids. (In the case of dairy and red meat, you'll be choosing lean, low-fat varieties so as not to overload on saturated fat.) You can also get protein through plants, especially grains, legumes, nuts and seeds, and soy foods (such as tofu and soybeans). Of these veggie sources, however, only soy is a complete protein. The rest are incomplete, so you need to combine them to get all the amino acids you need. But don't worry— there's no complicated food combining in the Active Calorie Diet. Foods that you naturally eat together—such as beans and rice, and peanut butter on bread—work together to make a complete protein. You don't even need to eat them at the same meal. So long as you eat all the essential amino acids within a day, you'll get all the complete protein you need.

The Active Calorie Diet makes getting all the protein you really need (not just what the RDA recommends) nearly effortless by simply changing the composition of your plate. You'll take away some of the

7 — GRAB-AND-GO PROTEINS

IN OUR EAT-ON-THE-GO CULTURE, most of the foods we choose for single-fisted consumption are highly processed and decidedly lacking in protein. It doesn't have to be that way. You don't have to carry around small zip-top bags of grilled-chicken strips to get your protein fix. Here are some super sources to take with you for your midday snack.

- **JERKY:** Jerky (beef or turkey) makes a great snack because it's low in fat, lean and savory, and high in the chewiness factor (look for lower-sodium varieties if you're concerned about the salt). You can find a wide variety of flavors, from teriyaki to barbecue. You can also find chicken and buffalo (and, in certain parts of the country, salmon) jerky. Jerky packs 10 grams of protein and about 100 calories per ounce.

- **ROASTED SOY NUTS:** Almonds, peanuts, and cashews are great. But let's face it: You can get burned out on the same nut mix. Try roasted soy nuts for a complete protein snack; for a little extra heat, try the wasabi-flavored ones. Each ¼ cup provides 6 grams of protein and 120 calories.

- **STRING CHEESE:** Not just for kids' lunch boxes, string cheese and other portioned cheeses such as The Laughing Cow Wedges or Mini Babybels are the perfect complements to an apple, pear, or bunch of grapes. At 80 calories and 7 grams of protein per stick, it's satisfying enough to carry you through to your next meal.

- **PROTEIN ISOLATE POWDER:** By itself, it's not high in chewiness, but in a fix it will help pump up your protein and give you a metabolic bump. Keep a Whey to Go protein powder in your pantry (or even in your desk at

pasta, rice, and bread; load up on vegetables, which also contain amino acids and contribute to that overall protein number at a very low calorie cost; and add lean meat, poultry, fish, or tofu. Many of the test panelists were surprised by just how easy (and tasty and satisfying) it was to incorporate more protein into their day. "Who knew I loved edamame?" says Melissa Shilling, 45, who lost more than 6 pounds in the first 2 weeks. "And the breakfast parfait is so big and filling. I love

work) for a quick protein fix. It comes in four flavors, mixes well with water, and delivers 16 grams of protein for only 70 calories.

• **BARS:** Protein bars are the perfect filling, portable snack to save you from a desperate trip to the vending machine or drive-thru station. Pick up bars that are about 200 calories each, such as Luna Protein bars (190 calories, 12 grams protein) or Honey Stinger protein bars (190 calories, 10 grams protein), to stash in your pocketbook.

• **HARD-COOKED EGGS:** Eggs really are one of nature's most perfect portable foods. Packed with protein and antioxidants, they satisfy your hunger and improve your health. Try Eggland's Best Hard Cooked Peeled eggs for a no-muss, no-fuss snack or meal. Along with the usual protein punch, these edible orbs also deliver 10 times more vitamin E and three times more omega-3 fatty acids than other eggs.

• **FAT-FREE OR LOW-FAT MILK:** It's the perfect pre- or postexercise snack. You can stock up on small containers of shelf-stable milk (such as Horizon's 8-ounce cartons); they don't even need to be refrigerated. Two cups deliver more than 16 grams of high-quality, filling protein that will satisfy your hunger and help keep you hydrated. In one study, women who had 18 grams of protein 20 minutes before strength training torched almost 9 percent more calories at rest 24 hours later than normal.[7] In an unrelated study, women who drank fat-free milk after they exercised lost 3½ pounds of fat in 4 months without doing anything else. By contrast, those who guzzled sports drinks (more on sugary liquids later) actually ended up gaining weight over the same 12-week period.[8] Choose fat-free or 1% milk to keep the protein without too much fat.

it!" Here's a look at some high-quality protein sources I'll be recommending in the Active Calorie Diet.

PROTEIN SOURCE (SERVING SIZE)	PROTEIN (GRAMS)
Steak (4 ounces)	34
Chicken breast (4 ounces)	26
Pork (4 ounces)	26
Tuna (4 ounces)	26
Salmon (4 ounces)	20
Greek yogurt, low-fat, plain (1 cup)	18
Yogurt, low-fat, plain (1 cup)	13
Eggs (2)	12
Tofu (4 ounces)	11
Lentils (½ cup)	9
Peanut butter (2 tablespoons)	8
Cheese (1 ounce, or 1 slice)	7
Nuts (1 ounce)	7
Pasta (1 cup)	7
Mixed vegetables (⅔ cup)	2

Carbs: Thermic Effect, 10 to 30 percent

Before you start reading this section, take an imaginary eraser and wipe your mental slate completely clean of everything you've heard about carbs during the past 10 years. Fat may have been unfairly demonized for a long time, but carbohydrate is hands down the most widely misunderstood macronutrient.

The Active Calorie Diet doesn't demonize carbs. Far from it. You need carbohydrates to keep your body moving. Carbs are energy. Your body turns them into glucose (blood sugar) and puts them into your muscles (glycogen) to burn when you walk, play, run around with your kids, and generally live your life. Your brain—command central for your thoughts, moods, actions, and metabolism—burns carbs and carbs alone. That's why you get grumpy and fuzzy brained if you don't eat enough. The problem is, too many of us have a woefully narrow definition of what carbs are and where they come from.

Somewhere along the line, "starch" became synonymous with "carb." While it's true that spaghetti, muffins, pancakes, and bagels are indeed carbs, they're not the only or necessarily the best sources. Many (though not all; more on that in a little while) starchy carbs set the stage for overeating. Remember that bit about your brain operating on carbohydrates? Your brain loves a quick fix, and quickly digested, starchy carbs are like FedEx to the brain. When you eat a scoop of pasta, your body quickly turns those carbs to sugar and delivers them to your cells very rapidly, which makes your brain happy and leaves you wanting more, even though you're not really hungry. In short, they make it pretty difficult to tune in and listen to what your body needs. In addition, because they shoot into your system so quickly, they're not very "active" in your digestive system and do little to bump your calorie burn. Instead, they rapidly shuttle into storage, where they become body fat.

The good news is, there are several types of Active Calorie carbs. The first and most healthful are fruits and vegetables, which are rich in carbohydrates but tend to be lower in calories and higher in fiber, so they digest more slowly and have a much higher thermic effect (about 20 percent). If you look at the Active Calorie Plate, you'll see that you'll be eating about half your meals in the form of fruits and vegetables. This will also ensure that you get as much fiber as you need to stay full, satiated, and healthy. I recommend that women get at least 25 grams of fiber and men get 38 grams each day. But again, no counting necessary. By simply following the meal plans and picking and choosing from the dozens of metabolism-raising foods in the Active Calorie lists, you'll automatically get all the dietary fiber you need.

Another benefit of these fiber-rich carbs is that you're much less likely to plow through so many strawberries and string beans that you end up with more fuel than you need. Vegetables are so rich in Active Calories (along with vitamins, minerals, and other disease-fighting phytochemicals and antioxidants) that the Active Calorie Diet gives you a free pass to eat as many as you want without counting them. Fruits are a bit higher in sugar, so you can overdo them if you're not careful. But you can still have fruit with every meal. If you're not yet in the habit of making fresh produce part of every meal, the Active Calorie Diet will help by placing them front and center on your plate every time you sit down to eat.

Other Active Calorie carbs include hearty, fiber-rich whole grains and beans. I especially like brown rice, barley, oats, and rye, because they contain a special type of fiber (called resistant starch) that is not easily digested, so they take up space in your digestive system, helping you feel full sooner and avoid the bingeing fate brought on by most other easily digested starchy carbs. These foods also have a high thermic effect and are particularly good at burning fat. When these undigested starches get to your large intestine, they ferment, in the process generating a fatty acid called butyrate, which appears to hinder your body's ability to burn carbohydrates. With your carb stores unavailable, your body turns to stored fat for fuel. In one study, researchers found that men and women who swapped just over 5 percent of their total carbs with resistant-starch–rich carbs burned 20 to 30 percent more fat after their meal.[9] As if that weren't enough, these hearty foods may even help quiet hunger hormones.

A bonus benefit of getting your carbs from whole grains and beans is that these foods also contain amino acids. So when you combine them in a dish, such as beans and brown rice, you'll get not only the metabolism-revving effect of resistant starch but also, since those foods create a complete protein, a bonus bump in thermic effect from that macronutrient. That's the real power of the right mix of Active Calories.

Sure, you know there are carbs in cereal and cake. But widen your horizons and you'll find dozens of Active Calorie carbs in some surprising places. You'll also save many hundreds of unwanted and unnecessary calories. One softball-size cup of spaghetti will set you back about 220 calories. An equally large portion of cooked veggies comes in at about 30. That saves 190 calories while adding countless antioxidants, vitamins, minerals, and other disease-fighting phytonutrients. Plus, the fiber in fruits and veggies helps fill you up faster. Here's a list of some of my favorite hearty Active Calorie carbohydrate sources. (Note: Although sweet potatoes are technically a vegetable, I'll be treating them as a starch because of where they fall on the Active Calorie Plate.)

VEGETABLES (SERVING SIZE)	CARBS (GRAMS)
Succotash, cooked (1 cup)	47
Sweet potato, baked with skin (1 large)	44
Winter squash, cooked (1 cup)	30
Peas, cooked (1 cup)	25
Parsnips, cooked (½ cup)	15
Onions, raw (1 cup, diced)	14
Artichoke, cooked (1 medium)	13
Collard greens, cooked (1 cup)	12
Pumpkin, cooked and mashed (1 cup)	12
Turnip, cooked and mashed (1 cup)	11
Green bell peppers (1 cup, diced)	10
Beets, cooked (½ cup)	8
Carrots, cooked (½ cup)	8
Tomatoes, raw (1 cup, diced)	8
Zucchini, cooked (1 cup)	8

Brussels sprouts, cooked (½ cup)	7
Eggplant, cooked (1 cup)	7
Kale, cooked (1 cup)	7
Spinach, cooked (1 cup)	7
Sweet corn, cooked (1 ounce)	7
Swiss chard, cooked (1 cup)	7
Broccoli, raw (1 cup, diced)	4
Celery, raw (1 cup, diced)	4
Leeks, cooked (½ cup)	4
Mushrooms, raw (1 cup, diced)	4
Radishes, raw (1 cup, diced)	4
Cabbage, cooked (½ cup)	3
Cauliflower, cooked (½ cup)	3

FRUIT (SERVING SIZE)	CARBS (GRAMS)
Mango (½ medium)	35
Pomegranate, raw (1 medium)	26
Pear (1 medium)	25
Pineapple (1 cup, cubed)	19
Peach (1 large)	17
Grapes (1 cup)	16
Honeydew (1 cup, cubed)	16
Nectarine (1 medium)	16

Cantaloupe (1 cup, cubed)	15
Kiwifruit (1 large)	14
Orange (1 medium)	14
Raspberries (1 cup)	14
Strawberries (1 cup)	11
Watermelon (1 cup, cubed)	11
Mandarin orange (1 medium)	8
Plum (1 medium)	8
Tangerine (1 medium)	8

Fats: Thermic Effect, 5 percent

Active fat. Sounds like an oxymoron, doesn't it? We have hated and avoided fat for so long in the United States, many people simply cannot view this vital macronutrient with anything but fear. Well, I'm here to tell you that it's no coincidence that our collective weight shot up as we slashed our fat consumption. Why? For one, because we were no longer full.

At 9 calories per gram, fat is the most energy dense of the macronutrients. We used to think that was a bad thing. Now we know better. That density makes your meals heartier, which in turn makes you feel more full with less food. When you eat fat, it can take hours before all the fatty acids work their way into your bloodstream. It also slows the emptying of carbohydrates from your stomach. That means your blood sugar stays more even, you don't get spikes and crashes in insulin, and you feel satisfied until it's time for your next meal. When you consider this, you can see that fat doesn't make you fat. Eating healthy amounts of fat is simply one of the best ways to curb hunger.

Fat has a pretty low thermic effect, but that doesn't mean it won't help raise your metabolism. Though your body doesn't do a lot of work chewing or digesting it, fat—particularly unsaturated fat—is essential for firing up your fat-burning metabolism. In a study of 101 men and women, Harvard researchers put half the group on a low-fat diet and half on a diet that obtained about 20 percent of its calories from mono-unsaturated fatty acids (MUFAs). After 18 months, the MUFA-eating group dropped 11 pounds and whittled about 3 inches off their waists, compared with their low-fat–eating peers, who shed only 6 pounds.[10] Because your body burns fat during aerobic exercise, eating a diet that's a little richer in healthy fats will also help you exercise longer and—guess what?—burn more fat! Research finds that men and women who eat diets higher in fat can run and ride bikes longer before tiring out than those who eat low-fat, high-carb diets.

By following the Active Calorie Diet and its emphasis on hearty and chewy proteins (such as fish, lean meats, soy foods, poultry, and dairy), you will automatically be eating a diet that gets about 25 percent of its calories from fat. As you'll see, there is no special partition for fat on the Active Calorie Plate, since fat is generally integrated into the other foods on the plate. As with carbohydrates, however, the quality of your fat is even more important than the quantity. As you likely know, fat comes in a variety of forms: saturated fat, unsaturated fat, and trans fatty acids.

Saturated fats are those found in animal products such as meats, dairy foods, and eggs, as well as certain plant foods like coconut and palm kernel oil. You can spot a saturated fat because, like butter or lard, it is solid at room temperature and melts when heated. Contrary to what people used to think, saturated fats are not all bad. In fact, a certain amount of saturated fat is healthy, even necessary. Saturated fatty acids help maintain your cell structure, produce hormones, build a healthy nervous system, and strengthen bone. I'm not suggesting that you live on steak and eggs, but I am saying that both have a prominent place in the Active Calorie Diet, and with good reason.

Unsaturated fats include MUFAs and polyunsaturated fatty acids (PUFAs); both types are liquid at room temperature but begin to solidify when you chill them. MUFAs come from olive oil, nuts, seeds, and avocados, while PUFAs come in two forms: omega-6 and omega-3. Your body can't make or store either type, so you have to include them in your diet on a regular basis. Omega-6s, which are found in vegetable oils like corn, sunflower, safflower, soybean, and cottonseed, are plentiful in most processed and fast food. As a result, we tend to eat more of these than we need or is healthy. Omega-3s are not so easy to come by. They're found in small doses in nuts and some plants, but hands down, the best source of omega-3 fatty acids is fish, especially the cold-water variety like mackerel, sardines, and wild salmon. Omega-3s are instrumental in nearly every function of your body, from generating healthy cells to forming the building blocks of your brain and eyes. They turn genes on and off; help cells communicate with one another; fight infection; and, maybe most important, quell inflammation.

Though both saturated and unsaturated fats are allowed in the Active Calorie Diet, the preferred fat sources for maximum metabolism revving are MUFAs (which come from plants and the plant oils you cook with, among other food sources) and omega-3s. These fats contain special molecules that help your body shuttle more fat into your cells' mitochondria (the fuel-burning, energy-producing furnaces) to be used as fuel. So when you eat foods rich in MUFAs and omega-3s, more fat gets shuttled into cells, and your thermogenesis (calorie-burning) and metabolic rate goes up.

As mentioned earlier, fat is very energy dense, so a little—even of the healthy variety—still goes a long way. You can't eat it with abandon. Here are what healthy portions of MUFA-rich foods look like.

- **Nuts and seeds:** Break free from the typical peanuts and peanut butter. Try pecans, pine nuts, almond butter, and tahini (sesame paste). A serving size is 2 tablespoons.
- **Olives:** Look for black, green, or mixed, or blended in a spreadable tapenade. A serving is 10 large olives or 2 tablespoons of tapenade.

{ carole stieg }

Reinventing Herself from the Corner Booth at the Bar

AGE: 60

POUNDS LOST:
7.4

INCHES LOST:
7 1/2 including 2 off her thighs

CAROLE STIEG likes life on the simple side. She, her husband, and friends have their own little booth down at the local bar. "That's just the way it is," she says with an easy shrug and a smile. But creeping weight gain and low energy left her wanting to make some healthier changes. For Carole, the Active Calorie answer was about what she needed to add in, not take away from, her life. "I'm not a big veggie eater, but I've discovered ways to eat more without making any real sacrifices in the dishes I love. I order the steak salad at the bar, which is great." For heat, Carole says, "I started carrying cinnamon sticks with me to add a zip to my coffee. It's easy!" Since she eats out often, she also wanted to learn more about proper portions. She bought a food scale and measuring cup to weigh and measure a few dishes to see what proper portions looked like.

It worked like a charm. "I am pleased to have lost about 5 to 10 pounds in a pretty short time without making huge changes in my life. My clothes are fitting better, and I feel better. I'm not exhausted at the end of the day anymore, even when I have my three young grandchildren to watch! I'm thrilled."

- **Oils:** Olive, safflower, walnut, peanut, and flaxseed are all great. Cook with them, drizzle them, and eat them in pesto. One serving is 1 tablespoon.
- **Avocado:** Eat in guacamole. Or just slice and serve. One-quarter cup equals 1 serving.
- **Dark chocolate:** Must be dark or semisweet. Aim for ¼ cup, or about 2 ounces.

Fishing for omega-3 fatty acids may take a little more work, since the sources are scarcer in our usual diets. I recommend aiming to average about 1 gram a day. Here's how some common sources stack up. The easiest way, as you can see, is choosing fish a few times a week for your chewy and hearty Active Calorie protein.

FOOD	OMEGA-3S (GRAMS)
Herring (3 ounces)	1.9
Salmon (3 ounces)	1.9
Tuna (3 ounces)	1.5
Anchovies (2 ounces)	1.2
Sardines (2 ounces)	1.2

The only fats that aren't allowed in the Active Calorie Diet are trans fatty acids, or trans fats, the man-made kind found in commercial cakes, frostings, shortenings, and some processed foods. As you'll learn in Chapter 4, these fats, which go by the names "hydrogenated oils," "partially hydrogenated oils," and "vegetable shortening," are not only bad for your heart; they also may make you fat. Primate studies have found that monkeys fed a diet high in trans fats (but not excess calories) packed on four times as much weight (much of it in their bellies) over a 6-year span as a similar group of monkeys that ate the same calories with healthier fats.[11]

The good news is that the Active Calorie Diet is naturally low in trans fats, and food manufacturers are steadily removing them from our food supply. But it's still wise to read the labels if you buy a lot of packaged foods.

Liquid Calories: Easy Come, Easy Flow

The liquids you choose to wash down your meals with or to sip during other times of the day can fire up your weight loss efforts—or cause them to backfire. Too often, the choices that seem right, if not righteous, are anything but.

Take diet soda. A 7-year study of more than 1,550 men and women ages 25 to 64 found that for each can of diet soft drink consumed each day, a person's risk of obesity went up 41 percent.[12] What's going on? The body is not so easily tricked. Researchers believe that when your taste buds taste something sweet, your body has an expectation of calories that will come with it and may actually trigger overeating until it gets what it expects. (Though studies have not been done, I suspect that this effect is also true for foods that contain artificial sweeteners.)

Now consider wine and other alcoholic beverages. A recent study of nearly 20,000 women found that participants who drank the equivalent of one or two glasses of wine per day gained fewer pounds than women who drank soft drinks or mineral water.[13] Though alcohol gets a bad rap, it can be a weight loss ally—if consumed in moderation. (Also beware of high-calorie mixers, like fruit juice and sodas, that are frequently high in added sugar or other Couch Potato Calories.) Scientists theorize that the livers of regular imbibers break down alcohol by turning the extra energy into heat, not fat. So if you drink 100 calories from chardonnay (or your favorite cocktail), it will mostly be burned off, while the same 100 from a cupcake will transform into fat.

Is that license to crack a bottle of cabernet and go to town? No. But

EASY ON THE ALCOHOL

ALCOHOL IS NOT OFF-LIMITS in the Active Calorie Diet. In fact, in moderation—that's a drink a day—it fits right in as an Active Calorie food. But you need to be very careful with this one because too much beer, wine, or spirits tips the scales into the Couch Potato category by lowering inhibitions and triggering overeating. It's important to be mindful of this when eating out and the first question the server asks is "Can I get you something to drink?"

In a study of more than 37,000 men and women, researchers found that those who drank about one drink per day 3 to 7 days a week had the lowest BMI (body mass index, a measure of body weight according to height), while those who frequently consumed the highest quantities of alcohol had the highest BMIs.[14]

Not only can alcohol itself (and common mixers in alcoholic drinks) carry a heavy calorie load, but when you drink too much alcohol, you lower your blood sugar, which leaves you ravenously hungry and primed for a Couch Potato Calorie binge. (Why do you think pub food is notoriously high in starchy carbs? Fries, loaded potato skins, and fried cheese, anyone?) If you can't stop at one, it's probably better to have none.

it's food for thought about your beverage selection. I believe that well-chosen fluids—including tea, milk, coffee, and, yes, even wine—can help crank up your weight loss. The Active Calorie Diet takes advantage of those liquid jolts. Break out of the soda rut and pour some of these into your daily cup.

- **Green tea:** A cup of brewed green tea can boost your fat metabolism by 12 percent, according to Japanese research. That's because tea is brimming with thermogenic (metabolism-raising) ingredients such as caffeine and fat-burning natural antioxidants called catechins. A recent review study found that these ingredients can increase daily calorie burn by about 72 to 96 calories (the amount in a chocolate chip cookie).[15] Green tea is the best source of catechins, but Earl Grey or another favorite black tea will give you a metabolic bump as well. If it's been a while since you tried green tea, give it another go. Long gone are the days when all you could find were grassy-tasting bitter greens. You can find sweet, flavorful varieties that include fruit, ginger, and other flavors. A few of the test panelists fell in love with tea and took to brewing enough to sip throughout the day.

- **Coffee:** Your morning cup of coffee (that's plain or with just a little cream and sugar, not a grande mocha) gets things off on the right foot. Caffeine is a central nervous system stimulant, so your daily java jolts can boost your metabolism by 5 to 8 percent—about 80 to 128 calories a day.[16] But remember that flavored syrups and whipped cream can add more than 100 calories and easily erase that deficit.

- **Wine and other alcoholic beverages:** As mentioned above, wine (or any alcohol) can be a fat burner. Just remember that moderation is very important here. Too much alcohol lowers inhibitions and leads to overeating. And many cocktails are made with high-calorie mixers like fruit juice or soda. Plus, too much alcohol can harm your liver (among other unhealthy effects). Stick to no more than one drink a day.

- **Sparkling water (flavored or plain):** Water is not exciting, I know. But it really does work for weight loss, and there are many varieties of naturally flavored sparkling waters to give soda lovers their fizzy-bubble fix. It's also an easy way to take off a few pounds. A study of 240 women dieters showed that those who swapped their sweetened drinks with water lost an average of 3 pounds more than those who didn't. Those who drank more than 4 cups a day lost an additional 2 pounds, compared with those who drank less.[17]

- **Fat-free or low-fat milk:** It's not just for kids. Milk is good for grown-ups, too, especially those looking to lose a few pounds. According to a study published in the *American Journal of Clinical*

Nutrition, women who drank fat-free milk (I like 1%) at breakfast ate about 50 fewer calories at lunch than they did on days when they sipped the same number of calories from orange juice or other fruit juice. Another study reported that women who drank 1% milk after exercising lost 3½ pounds of fat in 12 weeks, while their counterparts who sipped sugar sports drinks ended up gaining weight![18] The Active Calories from protein and the healthy fat in milk simply leave you more satisfied and help make muscle, too.

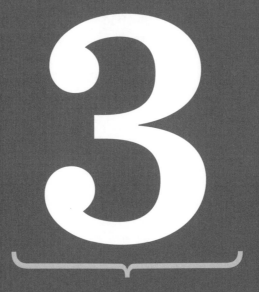

3

Lose More:
The CHEW Factor

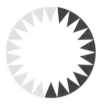

nergy. The heart and soul and foundation of the Active Calorie Diet is all about energy—how to get more from your food, how food can give you more, and how you can eat in a way that not only gives you plenty of energy but also burns energy. It's about making your body work with the food you eat and making your food really work for you. If you imagine your metabolism as an energy-producing (and calorie-burning) furnace, Active Calorie foods are like propane-doused briquettes. They get the fire started and keep it burning hot for hours on end.

The fancy name for this process, as mentioned previously, is the thermic effect. Foods that are rich in Active Calories have a high thermic effect—they make your body use lots of energy to process and digest them. Simply by eating, you raise your metabolism and trip the weight loss switch. Specifically, there are four types of Active Calories, based on the thermic effect of food science from Chapter 2. I believe you should eat all four of these each and every day, including at least two at every meal and one at every snack.

They are as follows:

C-hewy

H-earty

E-nergizing

W-arming

The bulk of your meals should be made of chewy and hearty foods, with energizing and warming spices, seasonings, and foods included as much as possible.

Chewy Foods

These are the Active Calories that make your body work right off the fork. It's a job for your body to process, digest, and use them—in other words, these are the foods with the biggest thermic effect, as we just learned. They include lean meats, nuts, and fiber-rich foods, as well as fresh fruits and vegetables. Whenever possible, choose food as close to "whole" as possible—e.g., a tuna steak instead of canned tuna, an apple instead of applesauce—to increase its chew factor. It makes a bigger difference than you'd think. Studies show that eating ground meat reduces the cost of digestion by nearly 13 percent.[1] So eating a medium-rare steak will provide far more Active Calories than wolfing down a burger.

You'll notice that some Active Calorie foods will appear in more than one category. For instance, fruits and vegetables are both chewy and hearty. Similarly, although nuts get most of their thermic effect from their chewiness, they also contain healthy fats that contribute to satiety (the filling feeling that's key to hearty Active Calories). That's why, on the Active Calorie Plate, which you will learn more about in Chapter 5, I make a point of defining the types of chewy and hearty foods you should be putting in each partition (that is, a little more than a quarter of your plate should come from chewy protein, about half from chewy and hearty fruits and vegetables, and a little less than a quarter from hearty grains). As you might imagine, the more Active Calorie categories a food falls into, the bigger your metabolic boost.

"I've learned to love pistachios," says panelist Cherry Semple White, who lost 4½ inches off her waist. "I buy them in the shell, so I have to work to open them, and I'm not just mindlessly shoveling them into my mouth. It takes me longer to eat them. I appreciate them more because I'm actually paying attention to eating them. And I eat fewer because I'm satisfied with less."

As a bonus, I've also included gum—though not a food—in the chewy category. Though I would never recommend incessant gum chewing, a few sticks a day can help you shed pounds. In a study of 35 men and women, researchers from the University of Rhode Island found that when the volunteers chewed gum for an hour in the morning, they ate 67 fewer calories later in the day. What's more, they felt less hungry and burned 5 percent more calories than on days they didn't chew gum.[2]

Hearty Foods

You want your food to have some substance so it's filling and satisfying. Hearty Active Calories help you lose weight by increasing your satiety, taking up more room in your belly (compared with other foods that have the same number of calories) and leaving less room for unnecessary second helpings. They include fiber-rich and fluid-rich foods as well as fluids themselves.

Fruits and vegetables are my favorite form of hearty Active Calories because they often have lots of fiber and are heavy with fluid, so they're also very filling. And, depending on how you prepare them, vegetables can be both chewy and hearty. Raw carrots (I love baby carrots!) are a great example. Raw carrots take lots of energy to chew—40 percent more than cooked carrots, in fact. So eating veggies raw or cooking them so that they're still crunchy can increase their thermic effect.

(continued on page 40)

{ bill ankrom }

Man with a Plan

AGE: 39
POUNDS LOST:
12.4
INCHES LOST:
$7^{1}/_{4}$ including 4 off his waist

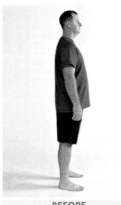

BEFORE

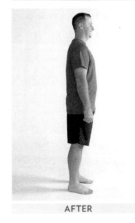

AFTER

LIKE SO MANY of my clients, test panelist Bill Ankrom knew what he needed to do. He just couldn't seem to do it. Every evening was a random array of eating and drinking, from the time he got home to the time he called it a night. "I'd be nibbling on pretzels, drinking beer, picking at leftovers, and eating something or other pretty much constantly," he recalls. Social situations were even worse. Family parties, church functions, and picnics pretty much did him in. Unlike other panelists, who embraced the opportunity to learn new dishes with the Active Calorie recipes, Bill had no interest. He was "content" with the foods he enjoyed; he just needed to learn how to manage his intake better—to activate his existing diet. I'm happy to say he was a fast learner.

Now 13 pounds lighter, Bill reports that his new eating habits are getting easier, and he's more motivated to learn about creating an Active Calorie Plate because he's losing so much weight. What worked? Drinking more water, for one. Bill likes beer. So he bought low-calorie beer, like Yuengling Light and MGD 64, for football Sundays. Then he was sure to drink equal amounts of water. He also did well simply thinking about his food choices ahead of time. Bill made sure he had cereal bars in his desk drawer and smart Active Calorie snacks that were accessible so that he didn't show up to events hungry and vulnerable to temptation. "Just a little bit of preparation and

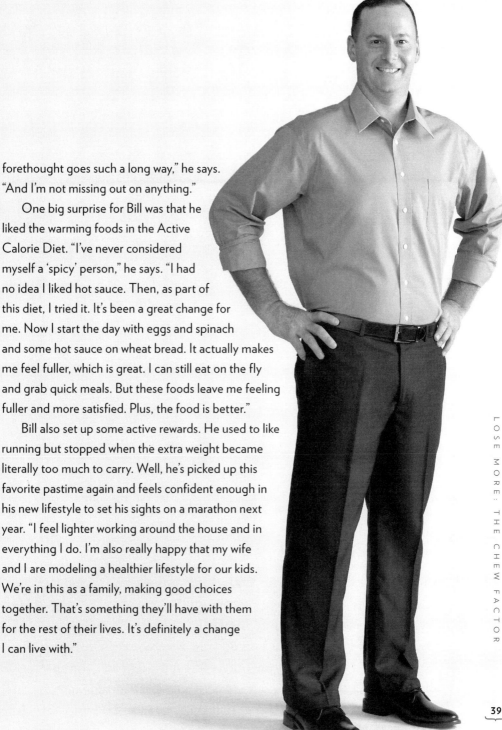

forethought goes such a long way," he says. "And I'm not missing out on anything."

One big surprise for Bill was that he liked the warming foods in the Active Calorie Diet. "I've never considered myself a 'spicy' person," he says. "I had no idea I liked hot sauce. Then, as part of this diet, I tried it. It's been a great change for me. Now I start the day with eggs and spinach and some hot sauce on wheat bread. It actually makes me feel fuller, which is great. I can still eat on the fly and grab quick meals. But these foods leave me feeling fuller and more satisfied. Plus, the food is better."

Bill also set up some active rewards. He used to like running but stopped when the extra weight became literally too much to carry. Well, he's picked up this favorite pastime again and feels confident enough in his new lifestyle to set his sights on a marathon next year. "I feel lighter working around the house and in everything I do. I'm also really happy that my wife and I are modeling a healthier lifestyle for our kids. We're in this as a family, making good choices together. That's something they'll have with them for the rest of their lives. It's definitely a change I can live with."

Whole grains, which are rich in fiber, also fall into this category. Many of the test panelists were surprised at how much fuller they felt simply by making the switch to hearty Active Calories. "Brown rice loaded with vegetables is so chewy and filling and satisfying," raves Suzanne Coglio, who lost 12 pounds. "I've been so used to white bread and white rice, I never realized how much more filling and really good other options could be."

I offer just a precaution or two for when you're choosing your fiber-rich hearty Active Calorie cereals. Fiber-rich foods, especially cereals, are a waist watcher's best friend, but beware the low-in-the-bowl syndrome it can cause. High-fiber cereals often come in dense, small pieces that can look like a pauper's portion when you pour the correct amount, leaving many people to serve up twice the serving size—and twice the calories. Look for fiber in flake form, like Kellogg's All-Bran Complete Wheat Flakes. They have 90 calories per ¾ cup, compared with the 140 you'd get from a similar amount of Bran Buds. Or use the Bran Buds as a topping to add crunch.

Remember to drink plenty. Drinking enough fluids makes every meal more hearty because it fills your tummy and expands the fiber to take up even more room. I like green tea because of its energizing effects. Carbonated water can help, too. Though it can have a very temporary bloating effect, it helps you feel fuller sooner, which will make you slimmer over the long term.

Energizing Foods

These calories fire up your central nervous system (and hence your metabolism). They include the metabolism-revving compounds caffeine and catechins. You'll find caffeine in coffee, of course, and black tea—just be careful not to load up your beverage with milk, cream, or sugar. And I don't recommend soda, even diet soda (more on that later). If you're not a java lover, no need to make yourself jittery by guzzling cups of joe. Green tea, as explained in Chapter 2, has very little caffeine but does contain high levels of metabolism-boosting catechins.

A study published in the *American Journal of Clinical Nutrition* reported that men and women who drank iced green tea packed with 690 milligrams of catechins (about three mugs' worth) lost more than 5 pounds, mostly from fat, and more than an inch off their waists over a 12-week period—double the loss of those who drank a beverage with fewer antioxidants.[3] Previous research has shown that green tea extracts can raise resting metabolism about 4 percent or burn about 80 calories a day.[4] You can buy green tea packets that fit neatly in your purse. Just pour the contents into 16 ounces of water for a delicious, refreshing metabolism boost. "Tea has been a revelation for me!" says panelist Camilla Monti, who dropped a dress size. "I knew I should be drinking more fluids, but I really don't like water. Now I can experiment with all these great teas that taste so good and are good for me, too!"

More good news: Since dark chocolate contains both catechins and caffeine (milk chocolate is not a good source of catechins), it also falls into this category. Obviously, dark chocolate has some fat (healthy!) and calories, though, so stick to the portions recommended on page 29.

Warming Foods

Forget bland, sugary condiments and flavorings like ketchup, sour cream, and mayo. If you want to crank up the thermic effect of food and fully activate the calories from every meal, add some heat. Adding heat to meals gives your body a better calorie burn. You know how hot food makes you flush? That's because it's revving your metabolism. A new study from UCLA found that dieters taking capsaicin, the chemical that gives jalapeño chile peppers and other peppers their burn, doubled their energy expenditure for hours after eating, compared with a similar group who were pepper free.[5]

What's more, the metabolic flames you fan when you douse your sandwich with salsa seem to target fat specifically. In one Australian study of 36 overweight men and women, researchers reported that the volunteers burned more fat after a meal spiked with chile peppers than

BE A PEPPER

THE METABOLISM-REVVING INGREDIENT in peppers is capsaicin. You can feel it at work when your cheeks flush—or perhaps you even break a light sweat—during a spicy meal. Many of the test panelists were thrilled to discover how much they enjoyed kicking up their everyday meals with a little heat. And many reported feeling fuller sooner from a spicy meal than a bland one. "The heat from the pepper flakes helps you feel satisfied and continues to warm your stomach while the food is digesting," says Natalie Wingard, 42, who lost $7\frac{1}{2}$ inches. "I simply felt full and satisfied longer after every meal." Research shows that for the best thermogenic effect, it's best to eat a little heat every day, as the Active Calorie Diet recommends. Though hotter peppers do deliver a greater metabolic boost, new research shows that you needn't have a high tolerance for mouth burn to reap these extra calorie-burning benefits. Even milder peppers like poblanos contain compounds that help erase up to 100 calories a day by binding to nerve receptors and sending fat-burning signals to your brain.

Scientists score the heat in these fiery gems on what is called the Scoville scale, which simply measures a pepper's capsaicin content. The following is how popular peppers rank.

TYPE OF PEPPER	SCOVILLE HEAT UNITS
Bell pepper	0
Poblano	1,500
Tabasco sauce	3,750
Jalapeño	5,500
Chipotle	5,000 to 10,000
Serrano	25,000
Cayenne (ground)	40,000
Habanero	210,000
Bhut jolokia (hottest on earth)	1,000,000

after one that packed no heat.[6] Why? It comes back to capsaicin. This high-octane compound improves your body's ability to clear insulin—the hormone that triggers body-fat storage—from your bloodstream after a meal. In the study, the insulin levels of chile pepper eaters were also 32 percent lower after a spicy meal.

Not much of a pepper person? Other spices and condiments that leave a warm feeling in your mouth—like cinnamon, ginger, garlic, cloves, bay leaves, and mustard—help too. USDA researchers have reported that just ¼ to 1 teaspoon of cinnamon taken with a meal can send your metabolism soaring twentyfold.[7] Substitute cinnamon for sugar on your oatmeal and in your morning latte, and you'll not only save a couple hundred calories a week but also fire up your fat-burning. Plus, these warming spices and herbs inspire you to drink more. Drinking enough fluids helps you feel full sooner and keeps your digestive system working smoothly, both of which are important for weight loss and maintenance. As usual, just be sure you stick to no- or low-calorie beverages.

Finally, straddling the line between liquid and spice is vinegar, which adds a nice warming bite to any meal. I recommend including vinegar as part of the Active Calorie Diet, and not just on salads. Vinegar is especially good at slowing stomach emptying, so it can put the brakes on any starchy carbs you eat. Scientists at Arizona State University found that just 2 teaspoons of vinegar drizzled on a carb-heavy food (think french fries) reduced the glycemic response (how quickly the carbs shoot into the bloodstream) by 20 percent.[8] In a study of 175 overweight men and women, Japanese researchers found that those who drank 2 tablespoons of apple cider vinegar a day had significantly less body fat and slimmer waist circumferences after 12 weeks than those who didn't drink vinegar.[9] Scientists believe the acetic acid in vinegar turns on genes that produce proteins that help break down fat, so you're less likely to accumulate it.

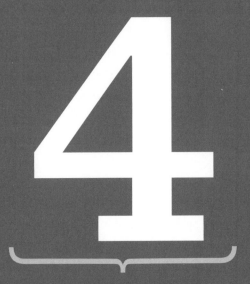

4

Lazy No More:
Turn Couch Potato Calories into Active Calories

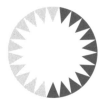

I believe in focusing on the positive—specifically, what you should eat rather than what you should not. But I'd be remiss here if I didn't spend some time talking about the foods you're better off avoiding, not just for weight loss but also for general health. These are foods that are rich in what I call Couch Potato Calories.

Walk through the aisles of any grocery store, and you'll find dozens and dozens of items that are so processed and/or filled with artificial ingredients that they barely resemble food. Not only does your body not have to do any work to eat or digest these foods, but it is also more likely to absorb every last calorie and stash it away as fat. That's why some of my clients struggle with their weight even when they're not eating too much food, because the lion's share of their calories consists of the empty, Couch Potato variety.

It's also why they feel so weighed down, both literally and figuratively. Their metabolisms are in a comatose state; the food they eat makes their blood-sugar levels plummet, leaving them with no get-up-and-go, and they're packing on pounds. One of the most striking benefits the test panelists noticed was that their energy levels went up almost immediately. In fact, all but one (who admitted that he did not follow the diet closely) of the 17 men and women on the panel reported big jumps in how energetic they felt. The first words out of one woman's mouth at the follow-up: "I have endless energy!" I guarantee you'll feel the same.

Some Couch Potato Calories are easy to spot. They are in the form of refined, sugary cakes and cookies and pastries, foods that you know aren't doing your waistline any favors. Others, like certain fruit juices, are less obvious. I've broken them down here so you know what to look for (and avoid) when you're filling your shopping cart.

The Pantry Stuffers: Sugar

These calorie sources are so refined and sugary that they take zero energy to digest, and because there's no protein or fiber standing in their way, they digest in the blink of an eye and shoot tons of sugar straight into your bloodstream. That sugar bomb trips a switch that spikes your insulin levels and quickly shuttles it all into storage as fat.

The first place to cut back is the sugar bowl. As I've noted, adding sugar to your coffee negates its energizing effect, and there's usually no need to sprinkle sugar on fruit, which is naturally sweet. And please note that this applies to all types of sugar! Brown sugar or raw sugar is not a more active type of sugar.

But it's likely that even if you never pick up the sugar spoon, you're consuming too much sugar in the form of processed foods. Most of these come in the "sweets" category, but not all. Check your cereal boxes as well as other packaged foods—even those you wouldn't expect, like bread and condiments such as ketchup—for added sugar. Note, too, that the package won't always say "sugar." These sweet pantry stuffers go by many names, most ending with "-ose," such as fructose, maltose, and sucrose. Added sugar also comes in the form of corn sweetener, molasses, syrup, honey, and fruit juice concentrates. Because so many foods are loaded with extra sugar, most Americans eat more than 22 teaspoons' worth (that's about 355 calories) every day. Spoon out that many teaspoons into a bowl (better make it a big bowl), and you'll be shocked at how much sugar you're unconsciously eating.

So how much sugar is okay? The obvious answer is as little as possible. But a little is unavoidable and will do you no harm. For a firm recommendation, I turn to the American Heart Association (AHA), which was concerned enough about the ill effects of added sugar that it issued a recommendation in 2009: Women should consume no more than 100 calories from added sugar per day, and men not more than 150 calories per day. Each gram of sugar contains 4 calories. So if you see that your morning muffin contains 15 grams of sugar, that's 60 extra pantry-stuffing calories you can (and should) live without.

While we're talking about sugar, I would be remiss if I didn't mention juice. Many of my clients consider juice a healthy elixir of sorts. In small doses, it's not bad for you; but it's also nowhere near as good for you as eating fruit. For one, many juices have added sugar. Even if they don't, fruit juice is by its very nature high in pure sugar (fructose), without any fiber to slow the surge of sugar into your circulation. Eight ounces of fruit juice, like pomegranate juice, packs 160 calories, more than a can of Mountain Dew. Sure, it's healthier. But it's still sugar, and unburned sugar will end up stocked in your fat stores. Instead, try pouring a 50-50 combination of juice and zero-calorie seltzer water to add fizz while shaving the calories in half.

What about artificial sweeteners like saccharin? As you'll find out shortly, it turned out that the promise of no-calorie sweeteners was too good to be true. So how can you best satisfy your sweet tooth? One word: fruit! Remember that the Active Calorie Diet includes three servings of juicy, sweet, whole fruit—that's one at every meal. Now, before you roll your eyes and say, "That's not what I meant," try changing how you prepare "nature's candy." It's true that many fruits, especially if not 100 percent ripe, have a little tang or tartness and may not satisfy that pure-sugar craving when eaten raw. But how about baked, grilled, or poached? Cooking fruit over high heat, such as on the grill, caramelizes (caramel—that's like candy, right?) the natural sugars, turning up the natural sweetness. Pineapple and mango are especially delectable. Baking apples and berries allows the flavors to mingle, and the simmering juices provide a perfect sweet "sauce." You can poach pears and other firm fruits in liquid (even a little brandy for a special treat), which enhances their natural richness. Strawberries with balsamic vinegar is one of my personal favorites. Remember also that a little dark chocolate (1 ounce, max) is a healthy way to get those energizing catechins and filling MUFAs (monounsaturated fats). What's more, Active Calorie living is about adjusting your plate to fit your life. You have that quarter of a plate where you can put your starch. Once in a while, if you choose, you can put some ice cream there (in a bowl, of course), substituting a sweet dessert for that starchy carb. I wouldn't do it every day, but on special occasions—sure. With all of these options, you can indulge that sweet tooth daily and still follow the Active Calorie Diet.

The Binge Brigade: White Starch

These are starchy, high-carbohydrate foods that you just cannot seem to stop eating once you start. Like sweets, high-starch foods such as pasta, white rice, and refined bread, muffins, and bagels can send your blood-sugar levels skyrocketing, triggering the same fat-storing insulin response as plain sugar.

These foods set you up for a binge in ways that can override even the most iron of wills. Scientists have discovered that high-carb (and high-fat) food activates your endocannabinoid (EC) system. If you break down that mouthful of a medical term, you'll see *cannabinoid*, which, you'll note, bears a remarkable resemblance to *cannabis*, or *marijuana*. What is marijuana known for? Munchies. It's a vicious circle that you can very innocently fall into without the use of any illegal drugs.

It works like this: You have cannabinoid receptors throughout your body, including your brain, gastrointestinal tract, and fat cells. They light up in the presence of blood sugar and insulin. When you swallow that spoonful of linguine, it sends sugar soaring into your bloodstream minutes later. Insulin gushes out to mop up the sweet spillage, and those receptors light up like an arcade pinball machine. This increases your endocannabinoids, which interact with other hormones to make you feel hungrier, leading you to eat more (usually more of the same stuff) and eventually pack on pounds. Over time, this overeating behavior can also lead to insulin resistance, which causes your body to become less effective at clearing blood sugar and ultimately can result in diabetes.

The solution for keeping your EC system calm? You guessed it: Active Calories. Foods that are high in fiber, water, and protein increase your sense of fullness, improve satiety, and slow down the flow of sugar into your bloodstream. Fruit (especially with a little chocolate) can satisfy your sweet tooth without causing an avalanche of food cravings.

The Fakers: Trans Fats and Artificial Sweeteners

You really can't outsmart Mother Nature. The fake fats and sweeteners that we engineered to let us have our cake and good health and waistline, too, have simply made things worse.

Let's start with one I mentioned earlier: trans fats. Although some trans fats are present in red meat and other animal-based foods, the ones that present a health hazard are the oils that have been engineered to make them firm, like vegetable shortening. For years we were told that these fats were actually a healthier alternative to other natural fats, like saturated fats. But it turns out that they're worse than even the worst natural fat. According to research, trans fats reduce the production of special structures inside your cells called peroxisomes, whose job is to shuttle fat into the mitochondria, or the cells' furnaces, so it can be burned for energy. Without adequate levels of peroxisomes, you simply can't burn as much fat as your body should or could, which explains why replacing natural fats with these fats did more harm than good for our collective health. It also explains why these fats seem to make us fatter. Be sure to read the ingredients, and look for terms like "partially hydrogenated" oils. Even if a product trumpets that it is trans fat free, there may still be small amounts in the product. Crackers are notorious

{ cherry semple white }

Breaking Binges

AGE: 58

POUNDS LOST:

5.6

INCHES LOST:

12$\frac{1}{4}$ including 4$\frac{1}{2}$ off her waist

CHERRY SEMPLE WHITE was a binge eater without really knowing it: "I would just sit in front of a movie with a bag of Oreos or a pint of Häagen-Dazs, and by the time it was over, it would all be gone. I didn't even feel stuffed, though I guess I should have."

Therein lies the pound-packing power of Couch Potato Calories. You can eat them—a whole lot of them—without even registering them, though your waistline sure does. It was Cherry's waistline—and her sister Carol, who did the program with her (see page 6)—that told her she needed to make a change.

After 4 weeks, she whittled her waist by 4$\frac{1}{2}$ inches. That's great news for Cherry, who has very high blood pressure, because belly fat is the type that really hurts your heart. "My cardiologist is very happy, and my sister helps keep me on track," she told us at the final weigh-in. "Mostly what I've learned is awareness."

When she does want some chips or ice cream, she measures out a serving to enjoy. "Since I'm not plowing through the whole bag, I take my time to enjoy every single chip," she says. "I know that a little treat here and there won't hurt because I'm eating well the majority of the time."

for having "zero trans fat" on the label because they don't contain enough trans fats per serving to have to list it, but the small amounts they do contain add up pretty quickly when you consider how many crackers you can consume. Best to avoid it entirely.

Ditto for artificial sweeteners. Back in the 1960s and 1970s, artificial sweeteners were supposed to save us from what was just the beginning of the weight problem in America. If we drank sodas with zero calories and put saccharin in our coffee, we'd save hundreds of calories and stay effortlessly slim, right? Wrong. As we saw earlier, diet-soda consumption has been linked to obesity, and sugar-free foods have certainly not solved our national weight problem. Whether it's because artificially sweetened foods make you crave more of the real thing or because they don't really satisfy your sweet tooth, so you tend to just keep eating and eating, they don't work for weight loss and are best avoided. If you use artificial sweeteners regularly, how about trying to cut down?

Another sweetener to avoid, as you've likely heard, is high fructose corn syrup (HFCS, sometimes called corn sugar or corn sweetener). There has been much heated debate among scientists, health officials, consumers, and the corn lobby about the potential ill effects of this processed sweetener. Some researchers believe that HFCS disrupts your body's hormonal feedback mechanism, which lets you know when you're full, so instead you feel hungry and continue eating, even when you've had plenty. Others claim that the modified sweetener actually encourages your body to store fat. A recent Princeton University study backs that suspicion.[1] The research team found that rats that drank water sweetened with HFCS gained significantly more weight than those that drank water sweetened with plain sugar, even when they drank the same number of calories. After 6 months, the rats that regularly drank the syrupy solution also had abnormally high increases in fat, especially dangerous belly fat, as well as a rise in triglyceride levels. More research is needed to confirm this effect, but since HFCS is not healthy and adds empty calories to your diet, I say there's no harm and more likely benefit in avoiding it, no matter what it's called.

The Impostors: Processed Foods

Beware processed foods that are advertised as the real thing but are really just a shell of themselves. Breaded chicken patties, chicken nuggets, and some processed burgers (including turkey burgers) are so ground up, pulverized, and fattened up with fillers that there's really no meat of substance left. Though veggie burgers are okay for the occasional picnic or quick lunch, I put those in this category as well. These "fake meat" foods tend to be highly processed, which puts them in the Couch Potato Calorie category.

Once you know what you're looking for, it's pretty easy to spot an impostor. Read your labels. Sometimes they'll actually have the word *processed* in the ingredients. If it doesn't say "processed," look for other key words indicating that the food you're about to eat may not be what it appears. These include *maltodextrin, mechanically deboned meat* (MDM), starches such as *modified potato starch, added flour, textured vegetable protein,* and other complicated, non-food-sounding ingredients. Be especially careful in the deli section, where you'll find some excellent choices (whole turkey breast) mixed with some highly processed Couch Potato foods, such as bologna and salami.

The best way to skirt impostors: Choose foods made with very few ingredients (aim for five or fewer) and ones that you recognize. Most manufacturers will make it clear that their hamburgers are 100 percent beef or their chicken sandwiches are from whole breast meat. Whole, unprocessed foods may cost a bit more, but the health and weight benefits will pay off in the long run.

Activate Every Calorie

For some people, the switch from Couch Potato Calories to Active Calories is relatively seamless and as simple as swapping a boxed burger for a homemade one or getting a fizzy liquid fix from flavored seltzer instead of soda. For others, this swap can be a sea change. When you're used to buying ready-to-eat foods that go from the microwave to your dinner plate in 45 seconds or less, you might find yourself wandering around the grocery store feeling as if there's suddenly no food to buy. That's certainly not true. But there are entire aisles in the supermarket stocked with foods that have little nutritional value.

I'll teach you the secrets to shopping for, preparing, and serving delicious Active Calorie meals in Chapter 6. In the meantime, rest assured that you don't have to give up all your Couch Potato Calories. Instead, learn how to "activate" those calories so that they take a little longer working their way through your digestive system and you get a little more energy burn out of them. Here's what you need to know to keep every calorie as active as it can be.

Prepare pasta Italian style: When you eat pasta in Venice, it is actually a chewy food, not the gummy mush that many of us pour onto our plates here. How do you get pasta perfectly al dente? Here are a few tips.

- Bring the water to a full, rolling boil before you pour in the pasta. If you put it in before you have a good boil, you risk getting a mass of soggy, starchy noodles.
- Go easy on the oil. I like to add a little oil to the water to keep the pasta from sticking. But limit it to a capful or you risk making the pasta soggy.
- Stir frequently so the pasta cooks uniformly and doesn't coagulate into one giant mass.
- Cook at the shorter end of the scale. If the box says 8 to 12 minutes, check the pasta at 7 to 7½ minutes. Spoon out a noodle and take a nibble. It should be firm but cooked, with no crunch. When it's done, drain immediately and serve.

Drizzle with vinegar: As mentioned in Chapter 3, vinegar is good at slowing down stomach emptying. In a 2005 study, Swedish researchers found that when men and women ate 2 tablespoons of vinegar with three slices of white bread (not that you'd be eating that much white bread in one sitting, but it's a good test), their blood-sugar levels were

COUCH POTATO
CALORIE WATCH LIST

THESE OFFENDERS ARE EASY to spot in a crowd. No food is ever forbidden. But keep these foods and similar ones to about 10 percent of your diet, and you'll have no trouble living an Active Calorie life. Like Active Calorie foods, there are some Couch Potato Calories that fall into more than one category.

THE PANTRY STUFFERS	THE BINGE BRIGADE	THE IMPOSTORS	THE FAKERS
• Candy	• Biscuits	• Bologna	• Cake-mix cakes and frostings (they often have trans fats)
• Candy bars	• Cookies, pie, and pastries	• Chicken nuggets	• Crackers
• Fruit punch and fruit juice cocktails	• Doughnuts	• Fruit punch and fruit juice cocktails	• Diet soda
• Soda	• French fries	• Hot dogs	
• Sweetened cereal	• Ice cream	• Onion rings	
• Sweet tea	• Potato chips	• Pepperoni	
	• Sweetened cereal	• Salami	

23 percent lower than when they ate white bread sans vinegar.[2] When you order from the deli, have them douse a little oil and vinegar on your sub instead of mayo for more of an Active Calorie sandwich.

Eat a mixed bag: The Active Calorie Plate includes a balance of a variety of foods for a reason: It slows down digestion. Whenever you're faced with eating a meal that consists primarily of one macronutrient—say, a plate of spaghetti with a side of sourdough—think about Active Calorie foods that will make the calorie burn better. Garlic is one. Meatballs are another obvious addition. It's all about balance, balance, balance.

Time your carb binge: Go ahead and have that doughnut once in a while (like on a Friday). Just eat it early in the day instead of late afternoon or, worse, late night. Quick-burning carbs seem to spike insulin more when you eat them later in the day. So if you're going to have them, have them at the morning meal, then stick to Active Calorie foods later. When you eat them early on, you've also got the full day ahead of you to burn off those quick-burning calories through daily activity and exercise. It's not a license to have a pastry every day. But once in a while, I understand.

Take advantage of exercise: Get moving early and often! Take the tips in Chapter 9 and put them to use today. Exercise helps you use all calories (especially Couch Potato varieties) better. A single workout improves your insulin response for a full day. That's because exercise empties out the stored carbs in your liver and muscles and gives the new blood sugar you produce after eating somewhere to go. The more often you move throughout the day, the healthier your insulin response. Insulin helps control your blood sugar, energy levels, and appetite, so a healthy insulin response is key to weight loss and maintenance.

5

Plan More:
The 4-Week Active
Calorie Diet

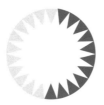

N ow that you have the full backstory on Active Calories and Couch Potato Calories, it's time to dig into the full 4-week Active Calorie Diet. Remember, this is not a short-term solution—it's a transformation of your relationship with food. For many of my clients, such as the ones you've met in this book so far, it's an entire life change. I know you're enthusiastic and raring to lose weight. But before I launch into the plan, I want you to remember a few things.

No one eats perfectly: You are going to "blow it" from time to time. I would actually prefer that you not look at it as "blowing it." That mind-set sets you up for "failure thinking": "I blew it with that doughnut. I might as well have these cookies . . . " Just accept that you're going to eat some Couch Potato Calories from time to time, and get right back on track with your Active Calorie eating for the next meal.

This is not a race: Again, I know you're anxious. But ultimately, trying to lose all the weight you can as quickly as you can will only backfire. This is about changing your relationship with food. That will take some time.

It is not always easy: Following the Active Calorie Diet should not feel laborious or difficult. And it should ultimately make you feel terrific, which makes everything easier. But I'll be honest—it won't always be a breeze. If you're not used to reading labels and cooking your own food, it may feel downright challenging at times. Try not to get too frustrated, however. Embrace it as a chance to learn and grow as you head down a healthier path.

Fine-tune; don't overhaul: These changes have to be sustainable. So if you've been living off of processed, boxed food for the better part of your adult life, you're going to put all that produce on the table and feel like a stranger in a strange land. This book is your guide. Start slowly, making manageable changes, and keep tweaking along the way.

Realize that weight loss consists of steps, not a slide: You will not necessarily lose pounds every week or the same amount of pounds every week, but that does not mean good things aren't happening. Quite a few of the test panelists commented on how their clothes were fitting better and they had much more energy before they saw numbers change on the scale. That's because as you get more active and eat more protein, you're putting on some lean muscle (which takes up less room than fat but weighs more) while you're losing fat. We are measuring success a number of ways here, and we're looking at the long term.

Your Active Calorie Plate

I've said it before and I'll say it again: I don't want you counting calories (though measuring your portions for the first month is very useful) unless you really want to. I'd rather have you honing your ability to "eyeball" the right amount of food. Plus, if you choose Active Calorie foods and create dishes that look like the ones presented here, there's no need to count. You'll be in the right range.

You've likely read diet recommendations before and been told to eat 60 percent of your food from one source and 20 percent from another. That's okay. But for many people it's meaningless because we don't think in terms of percentages when we dish out dinner. We put the food on our plates and eat. That's why I'm not asking you to calculate the thermic effect of each of your meals or telling you to eat precisely 40 percent chewy foods, 45 percent hearty foods, and 2 percent warming foods. Not only would it be a pain to have to track and calculate the calories, thermic effect, and composition of each food you eat, but it would also be impossible to really separate out different types of Active Calories.

Consider, for instance, a simple bowl of oatmeal made with milk and topped with nuts and berries. The oatmeal, a whole grain full of fiber, contributes to a high thermic effect. Plus, you'll get some protein from the milk and the nuts, which we also know gives a high thermic effect. But it would take quite a bit of math to figure out if that's a 20 percent or 25 percent thermic effect. Similarly, we know that the nuts are a chewy protein because they're a whole food that requires your body to do some work to chew and digest. But they're also a hearty food because their healthy fats help keep you full between meals.

The good news is, there's a much easier way to figure out what you need to eat in order to make sure you get enough Active Calorie foods. To keep the plan as easy to follow as possible, I like to provide visual cues. As one panelist told me, "I love the plate. The image is burned in my mind, so I can replicate it whether I'm at home, at a restaurant, or at friends' for dinner." One went so far as to copy it, blow it up, and hang it up in her kitchen! The following is what an Active Calorie Plate should look like. This, of course, is not a plate the size of a serving platter but, rather, a reasonable 9-inch dinner plate.

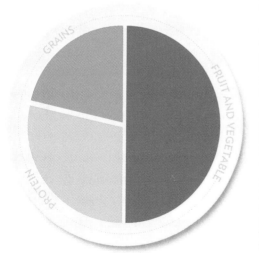

■ Fruit/Vegetable ■ Protein ■ Grains

A little more than a quarter of the plate should be chewy Active Calories from protein such as lean meat, skinless poultry, fish, soy foods, eggs, or low-fat dairy. This is about a palm-size amount of food, or about 4 ounces of cooked-weight food.

About half of the plate should be chewy and hearty Active Calories from fresh fruits and vegetables. This should be about two fist-size servings of fruits and/or vegetables.

A little less than a quarter of the plate should be hearty Active Calories from whole grain carbs such as brown rice, whole wheat pasta, potatoes, or tortillas (preferably whole wheat). A serving of these should be about the size of your fist, or 1 cup.

THE ACTIVE CALORIE BREAKDOWN

MOST PEOPLE DO WELL with having simple plate guidelines. But I know that there are some who really want to know the nutritional breakdown of their diet. If you're one of these people, this chart is for you. The purpose of the Active Calorie Diet is to provide a calorie level that encourages weight loss, divides the calories throughout the day, and provides a balance of foods in meals and snacks (though snacks don't always contain every element, since they're smaller) to keep your body energized and your brain satisfied. You don't have to count calories or grams, because the recipes do this for you. But if you decide

MEAL COMPOSITION

	WOMEN	MEN
Calories	1,500	1,800
Carb	50%	50%
Protein	25%	25%
Fat	25%	25%
Fiber	25 grams	38 grams
Fluid	90 ounces	125 ounces

CALORIES/MEAL

	WOMEN	MEN
Breakfast	400	400
Lunch	400	500
Dinner	500	700
Snack	200	200

A word about fat: Fat is an essential nutrient and an important element of the Active Calorie Diet. It does not have a special partition on the plate because fat is embedded in other Active Calorie foods, like fish, dairy, nuts, seeds, and even certain vegetables. When you eat foods that are rich in fat, like nut butters, avocado (guacamole), salad dressing, olives, and dark chocolate, be mindful of the portions on page 29.

In addition, for the biggest calorie burn, each meal should include at least one energizing or warming Active Calorie food. Teas, caffeine, that you want to know the breakdown that the meal plan is based on to help you prepare your own, the guidelines below provide a template for what the meals and snacks (or desserts) should look like. On most days, you should limit yourself to either a snack or a dessert of about 200 calories. But you'll see that in order to give you the most flexibility, I've also provided some 100-calorie snacks in Chapter 7. So if, on occasion, you're really craving both a snack and a dessert, stick to the 100-calorie options or have a "lunch" recipe for dinner so that you stay in the 1,500-calorie range for the day (1,800 calories for men).

WOMEN: MEAL NUTRIENT BREAKDOWN
(1,500 CALORIES PER DAY)

	BREAKFAST (GRAMS)	LUNCH (GRAMS)	DINNER (GRAMS)	SNACK (GRAMS)
Carb	50	50	69	27
Protein	25	25	25	10
Fat	11	11	14	5
Fiber	10	8	5	2

MEN: MEAL NUTRIENT BREAKDOWN
(1,800 CALORIES PER DAY)

	BREAKFAST (GRAMS)	LUNCH (GRAMS)	DINNER (GRAMS)	SNACK (GRAMS)
Carb	50	62	87	27
Protein	25	31	44	10
Fat	11	14	19	5
Fiber	15	10	11	3

and capsaicin increase daily calorie expenditure by about 5 percent apiece, or about 96 calories per day. Most of my clients find that they like adding heat to one or two meals daily, depending on their taste and tolerance (though remember that the meal doesn't have to be Tabasco hot). I like to see people drink 24 to 32 ounces of green tea, but if you choose a commercial iced tea, please be sure it's not loaded with sugar or high fructose corn syrup.

Finally, I would like you to drink two glasses of water with every

(continued on page 64)

{ suzanne coglio }

She Never Knew Good-for-You Food
Could Be So Good

AGE: 48
POUNDS LOST:
11.8
INCHES LOST:
$4\frac{1}{4}$ including $2\frac{1}{4}$ off her waist

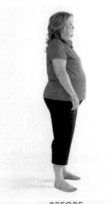

BEFORE

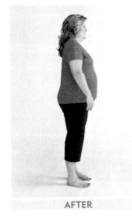

AFTER

WE'VE GOTTEN so far removed from real food, many of my clients are honestly stunned that they can eat well—really well—and still lose lots of weight. Such was the case with panelist Suzanne Coglio, who needed to buy new clothes by the end of her first month on the Active Calorie Diet because all of her old ones were too big. In her dieting life, losing weight meant cottage cheese; baked chicken; steamed, butterless broccoli; and plain, plain, plain, bland, boring, often tasteless foods.

"I loved having all these real food choices," she gushed at our final weigh-in. "It's opened up a whole new way of thinking about food and cooking for me! Before, I would have just eaten the plain chicken and the plain rice and really dreaded all of it. But these food combinations are so interesting and delicious that you never get tired of them. I was expecting more of the same old diet foods, which I really dread, and all I could think was *Wow, this is really good!* I was very surprised."

Even her husband, the cook in the family, jumped on board, if a bit reluctantly at first. "He's very used to white bread and buttered everything. So the first time he made my meal from the plan, he made himself some other food, just in case. Turns out he liked these meals so much, he went back for seconds. Even my teenage son liked it. We're all happily in this together."

If you're not used to eating healthfully, the toughest part is that initial shopping trip, notes Suzanne. "If you

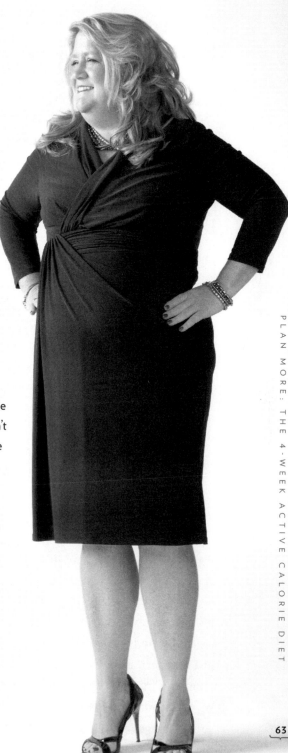

have a friend who eats healthy, you might want to take her along the first time. I spent a lot of time hunting for some of these foods at first. But once I knew where to find everything, it was much easier. We also did a little trial and error. Some wheat breads we liked; some we didn't. So I would encourage people to shop around and try different brands if they don't like something right away."

Now that she's seen the Active Calorie light, Suzanne is not going back. "This isn't a diet. I'm just finally eating healthier," she says, noting that her energy levels have nearly doubled and she feels far more confident than she has in years. "I'm in control of what I eat now. Sure, I still have sweets. But I'll have a couple pieces of fudge, not the whole box."

JUST FOR MEN

THE MEALS IN THIS BOOK follow the calorie and nutrient guidelines for women. Men need more calories because they're larger. Basically, guys, it's simple to adapt the plan for you: Just add 100 calories to lunch and 200 calories to dinner as follows:

100-CALORIE LUNCH ADDITIONS

8-ounce glass fat-free milk

2 slices reduced-fat American cheese

3 slices thinly sliced turkey breast

1/2 cup cottage cheese

1/2 cup edamame

8-ounce can vegetable soup

1/2 chicken breast, about 4 ounces

1 tablespoon peanut butter

200-CALORIE DINNER ADDITIONS

3 ounces cooked-weight chicken, turkey, lean beef, or fish

1/2 cup beans (kidney, chickpea, navy, black, or cannellini)

2 tablespoons feta cheese

1/2 cup ground beef, ground turkey, or textured vegetable protein (TVP) (fake meat)

2 ounces cooked-weight chicken, turkey, lean beef, or fish plus 1 cup vegetables

meal. Adding fiber and protein when you're not used to it can cause some bloating initially. Water will help keep your digestive system flowing smoothly. What's more, it's a very easy way to lose weight. In one recent study, 48 overweight men and women dieters who drank two glasses (16 ounces) of water before their meals lost 15.5 pounds in 3 months (non–water drinkers lost 11).[1] More important, a full year later, the water drinkers continued to lose weight, while the nondrinkers started regaining.

As you embark on the Active Calorie Diet, keep in mind that weight loss is not just about the foods you put on your plate. Your mission is to create an Active Calorie lifestyle. When I say "active," I am not talking just about running or getting on the elliptical machine. In addition to choosing foods that are more active, I want you to infuse activity into your eating, your workday or at-home day, and your exercise. These small changes add up to a big difference in the long run, helping you get results faster. Because I know that all of this can be a lot to remember, for the 4 weeks of the Active Calorie Diet, I'm asking you to try just one Active Eating Habit and one Active Life Habit per day. You'll learn more about these simple tips for adding activity in Chapters 6 and 9.

In summary, here are the things you'll need to do on the Active Calorie Diet.

- Eat three meals (breakfast, lunch, and dinner) and a snack every day.
- Make sure each meal follows the Active Calorie Plate proportions (snacks and desserts may have only one type of Active Calorie).
- Have at least one energizing or warming food per meal (not including snacks).
- Drink two glasses of water with every meal.
- Do at least one Active Eating Habit and one Active Life Habit every day.

Active Calorie Grocery Shopping

To give you a taste of what you're in for, I've provided a simple shopping list of Active Calorie foods below. There are certainly more foods that could be on this list (essentially every fruit and vegetable you find in the produce section, for instance). My (and many other dietitians') advice: Shop the perimeter of the store first. That's where it stocks the fresh produce, meats, poultry, fish, dairy, grains, and other whole foods. Fill up your cart with these foods (keeping in mind that these foods are fresh, so they may need to be eaten or frozen that week). Then go through the interior aisles, where all the packaged foods are. Top off your cart with wholesome packaged foods like nuts, tuna fish, fresh sauces, spices, frozen fruit and vegetables, and other makings for healthful meals.

Throughout the next 4 weeks, you'll find yourself eating plenty of these Active Calorie foods. I've listed them here primarily so that you can learn to identify and enjoy them. I strongly recommend that you follow the 4-week diet to get started. Afterward you'll be able to create your own meals with confidence, using the foods from this list.

ACTIVE CALORIE PROTEINS

Beans, dry or canned

Beef, lean, such as sirloin, tenderloin, flank steak, tri-tip, or skirt steak

Cheese (low-fat cottage cheese, part-skim sliced cheese, The Laughing Cow Wedges or Mini Babybels, string cheese, reduced-fat shredded cheese, part-skim ricotta cheese, Parmesan cheese that you grate yourself)

Chicken, skinless white or dark meat

Edamame

Eggs

Fish, fresh, frozen, or canned

Ham

Milk, fat-free or 1%

Nuts in shell

Pork

Seeds

Shellfish

Soybeans or soynuts, roasted

Soy burgers, veggie crumbles, or textured vegetable protein

Turkey bacon

Turkey breast

Yogurt, preferably Greek (higher in protein)

ACTIVE CALORIE FRUITS

Apples	Grapes	Pears
Apricots	Mangoes	Pineapple
Bananas	Melons	Plums
Berries	Nectarines	Pomegranates
Cherries	Oranges	Tangerines
Clementines	Papayas	
Grapefruit	Peaches	

ACTIVE CALORIE VEGETABLES

Avocados	Celery	Spinach
Broccoli	Cucumbers	Squash
Cabbage	Mushrooms	Tomatoes
Carrots	Peppers	Zucchini
Cauliflower	Salad greens	

ACTIVE CALORIE GRAINS

Barley	Corn on the cob*	Potatoes, white or
Bread, whole wheat	English muffin,	sweet*
Brown rice	whole wheat	Tortillas (wraps),
Cereal, whole grain,	Grits	whole wheat
such as Kellogg's	Oatmeal	
All-Bran or	Pasta, whole wheat	
General Mills	Pita, whole wheat	
Fiber One		

ACTIVE CALORIE ENERGIZING FOODS

Coffee	Dark chocolate	Green or black tea
	(in moderation)	

ACTIVE CALORIE WARMING FOODS

Adobo powder	Cloves	Lemon pepper
or sauce	Cumin	Mustard and mustard
Bay leaves	Garlic and garlic	powder
Black pepper	powder	Red-pepper flakes
Cayenne	Ginger and powdered	Spicy salsa
Chile and hot	ginger	Vinegar
peppers	Hot paprika	
Cinnamon	Hot sauce	

* Although these are vegetables, they count as a grain on your plate.

Putting Together an Active Calorie Meal

In Chapter 7 you'll find almost 80 recipes for meals and snacks to launch you full swing into Active Calorie living. But to help you get an idea of what an Active Calorie Plate looks like, I've provided a few easy sample meals here, just putting together foods from the lists above. Many of the snacks focus on just one or two elements of the Active Calorie Plate, since the portions are smaller than the ones in your meals.

BREAKFAST

YOGURT AND CEREAL

ENERGIZING FOOD:
Coffee or tea

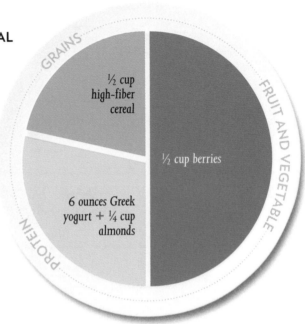

GRAINS

FRUIT AND VEGETABLE

½ cup
high-fiber
cereal

½ cup berries

6 ounces Greek
yogurt + ¼ cup
almonds

PROTEIN

CEREAL AND FRUIT

ENERGIZING FOOD:
Coffee or tea

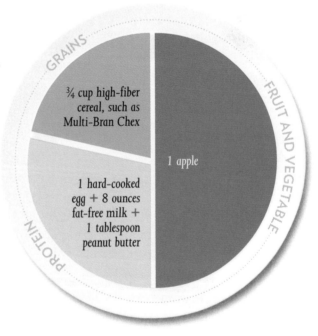

GRAINS

FRUIT AND VEGETABLE

¾ cup high-fiber
cereal, such as
Multi-Bran Chex

1 apple

1 hard-cooked
egg + 8 ounces
fat-free milk +
1 tablespoon
peanut butter

PROTEIN

OATMEAL

ENERGIZING FOOD:
Coffee or tea

WARMING FOOD:
Cinnamon to taste

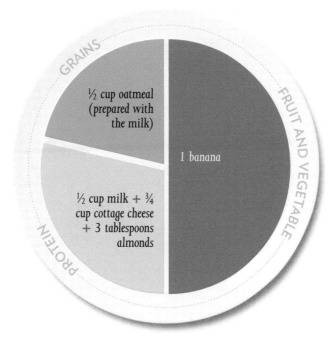

GRAINS

½ cup oatmeal (prepared with the milk)

FRUIT AND VEGETABLE

1 banana

½ cup milk + ¾ cup cottage cheese + 3 tablespoons almonds

PROTEIN

SCRAMBLED-EGG BURRITO

ENERGIZING FOOD:
Coffee or tea

WARMING FOOD:
Salsa

GRAINS

1 high-fiber tortilla, 6" diameter

FRUIT AND VEGETABLE

Green pepper + 1 orange

2 scrambled eggs + ¼ cup shredded reduced-fat Cheddar cheese

PROTEIN

HAM-AND-CHEESE SANDWICH

ENERGIZING FOOD:
Coffee or tea

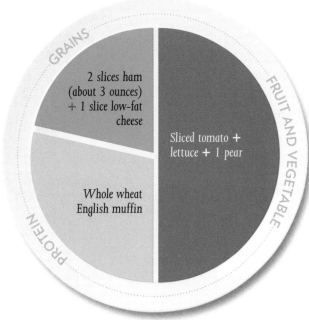

GRAINS

2 slices ham
(about 3 ounces)
+ 1 slice low-fat
cheese

Whole wheat
English muffin

Sliced tomato +
lettuce + 1 pear

PROTEIN

FRUIT AND VEGETABLE

WAFFLES

ENERGIZING FOOD:
Coffee or tea

WARMING FOOD:
Cinnamon to taste
(sprinkle on top)

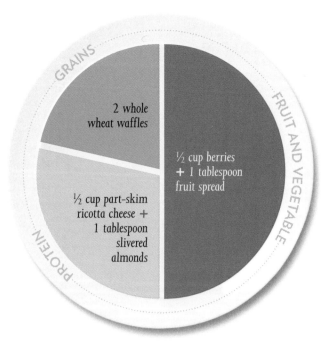

GRAINS

2 whole
wheat waffles

½ cup part-skim
ricotta cheese +
1 tablespoon
slivered
almonds

½ cup berries
+ 1 tablespoon
fruit spread

PROTEIN

FRUIT AND VEGETABLE

THE ACTIVE CALORIE DIET

LUNCH

TUNA PITA

WARMING FOOD:
2 tablespoons vinaigrette
(any kind)

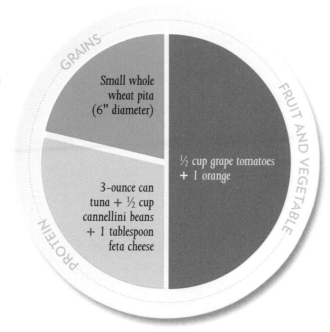

GRAINS

Small whole
wheat pita
(6" diameter)

FRUIT AND VEGETABLE

½ cup grape tomatoes
+ 1 orange

3-ounce can
tuna + ½ cup
cannellini beans
+ 1 tablespoon
feta cheese

PROTEIN

TURKEY WRAP

WARMING FOOD:
Jalapeño chile peppers
(fresh or jarred;
sliced or diced)

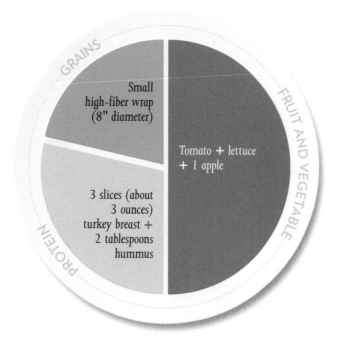

GRAINS

Small
high-fiber wrap
(8" diameter)

FRUIT AND VEGETABLE

Tomato + lettuce
+ 1 apple

3 slices (about
3 ounces)
turkey breast +
2 tablespoons
hummus

PROTEIN

TROPICAL SALAD

WARMING FOOD:
1 tablespoon balsamic
vinaigrette

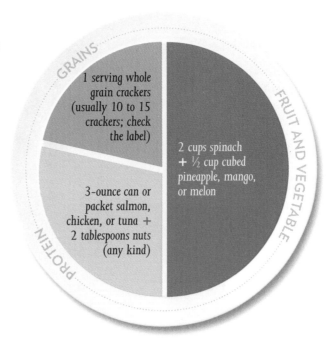

GRAINS

1 serving whole
grain crackers
(usually 10 to 15
crackers; check
the label)

3-ounce can or
packet salmon,
chicken, or tuna +
2 tablespoons nuts
(any kind)

PROTEIN

2 cups spinach
+ ½ cup cubed
pineapple, mango,
or melon

FRUIT AND VEGETABLE

OPEN-FACE
SANDWICH

WARMING FOOD:
1 tablespoon balsamic
vinegar and hot peppers
to taste

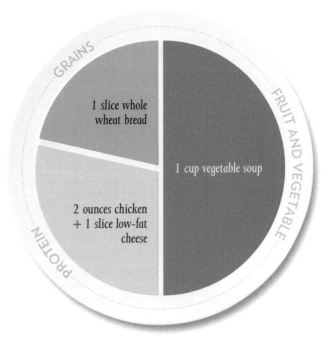

GRAINS

1 slice whole
wheat bread

2 ounces chicken
+ 1 slice low-fat
cheese

PROTEIN

1 cup vegetable soup

FRUIT AND VEGETABLE

THE ACTIVE CALORIE DIET

FAST-FOOD MEAL

WARMING FOOD:
Spices in chili

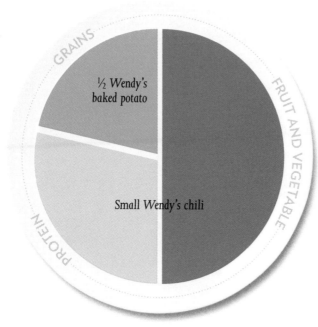

½ Wendy's baked potato

Small Wendy's chili

GRAINS

FRUIT AND VEGETABLE

PROTEIN

FROZEN MEAL

WARMING FOOD:
Cinnamon to taste
(to stir into the
Greek yogurt)

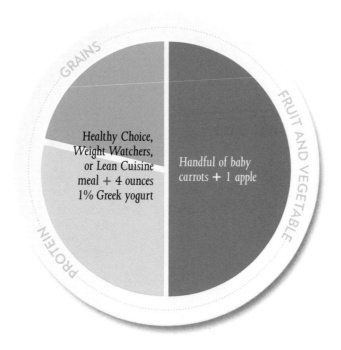

Healthy Choice,
Weight Watchers,
or Lean Cuisine
meal + 4 ounces
1% Greek yogurt

Handful of baby
carrots + 1 apple

GRAINS

FRUIT AND VEGETABLE

PROTEIN

DINNER

FISH

ENERGIZING FOOD:
Green tea

WARMING FOOD:
Hot pepper to taste

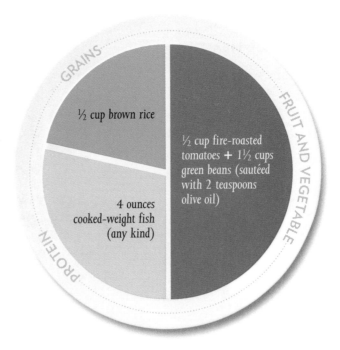

½ cup brown rice

4 ounces cooked-weight fish (any kind)

½ cup fire-roasted tomatoes **+** 1½ cups green beans (sautéed with 2 teaspoons olive oil)

GRAINS

PROTEIN

FRUIT AND VEGETABLE

PEANUTTY CHICKEN

ENERGIZING FOOD:
Green tea

WARMING FOOD:
Grated gingerroot (added to the vegetables)

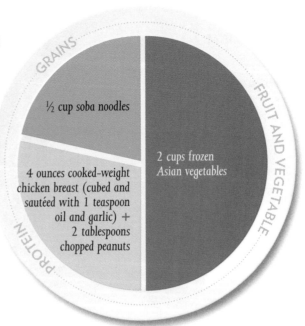

½ cup soba noodles

4 ounces cooked-weight chicken breast (cubed and sautéed with 1 teaspoon oil and garlic) **+** 2 tablespoons chopped peanuts

2 cups frozen Asian vegetables

GRAINS

PROTEIN

FRUIT AND VEGETABLE

BURGER OR STEAK

ENERGIZING FOOD:
Green tea

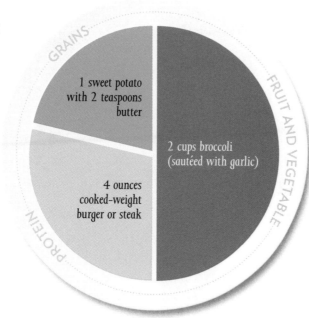

GRAINS

1 sweet potato
with 2 teaspoons
butter

FRUIT AND VEGETABLE

2 cups broccoli
(sautéed with garlic)

4 ounces
cooked-weight
burger or steak

PROTEIN

BEAN BURRITO

WARMING FOOD:
¼ cup salsa

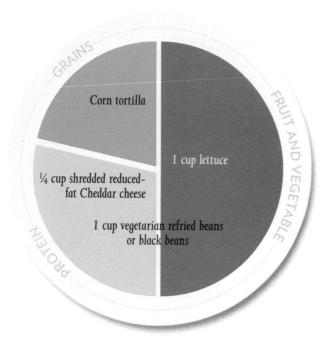

GRAINS

Corn tortilla

FRUIT AND VEGETABLE

1 cup lettuce

¼ cup shredded reduced-
fat Cheddar cheese

1 cup vegetarian refried beans
or black beans

PROTEIN

PASTA WITH SHRIMP

WARMING FOOD:
Red-pepper flakes to taste

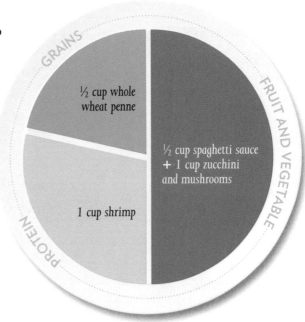

GRAINS

½ cup whole wheat penne

FRUIT AND VEGETABLE

½ cup spaghetti sauce + 1 cup zucchini and mushrooms

1 cup shrimp

PROTEIN

PORK AND POTATOES

WARMING FOOD:
Balsamic vinegar (to sprinkle on asparagus)

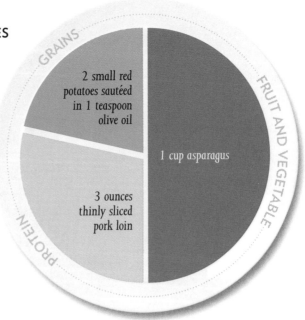

GRAINS

2 small red potatoes sautéed in 1 teaspoon olive oil

FRUIT AND VEGETABLE

1 cup asparagus

3 ounces thinly sliced pork loin

PROTEIN

SNACKS

YOGURT AND BAR

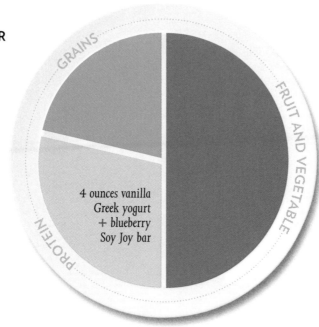

GRAINS

FRUIT AND VEGETABLE

PROTEIN

4 ounces vanilla
Greek yogurt
+ blueberry
Soy Joy bar

FRUIT AND CHEESE

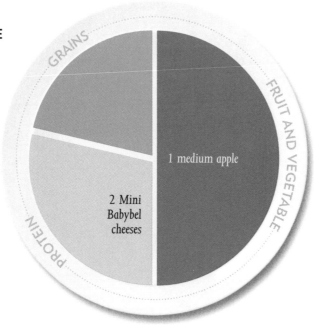

GRAINS

FRUIT AND VEGETABLE

PROTEIN

1 medium apple

2 Mini
Babybel
cheeses

TOMATO AND MOZZARELLA

WARMING FOOD:
Balsamic vinegar to taste

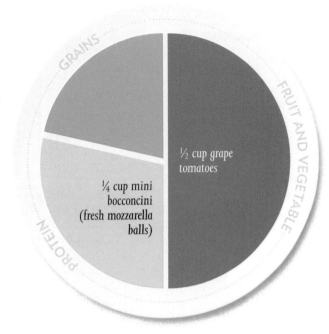

GRAINS

FRUIT AND VEGETABLE

½ cup grape tomatoes

¼ cup mini bocconcini (fresh mozzarella balls)

PROTEIN

POPCORN

WARMING FOOD:
Wasabi

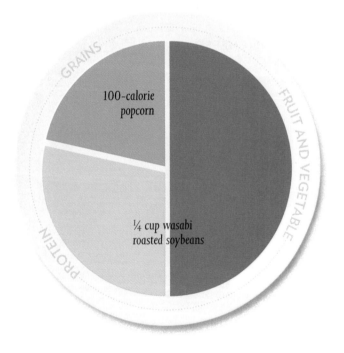

GRAINS

FRUIT AND VEGETABLE

100-calorie popcorn

¼ cup wasabi roasted soybeans

PROTEIN

GREEK YOGURT

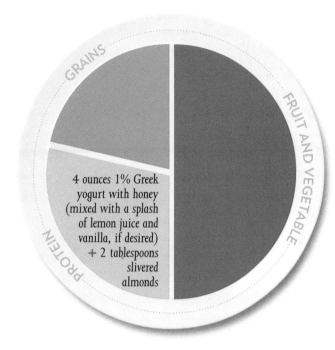

GRAINS

FRUIT AND VEGETABLE

PROTEIN

4 ounces 1% Greek
yogurt with honey
(mixed with a splash
of lemon juice and
vanilla, if desired)
+ 2 tablespoons
slivered
almonds

PROTEIN SHAKE

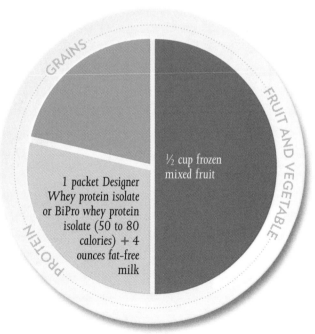

GRAINS

FRUIT AND VEGETABLE

PROTEIN

½ cup frozen
mixed fruit

1 packet Designer
Whey protein isolate
or BiPro whey protein
isolate (50 to 80
calories) + 4
ounces fat-free
milk

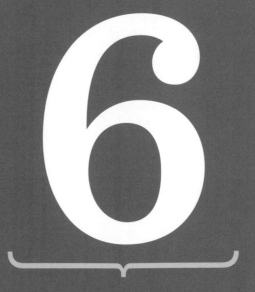

6

Create More:
The Active Calorie Kitchen

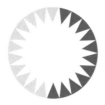

Have you ever watched *Iron Chef*? Or Anthony Bourdain's *No Reservations*? Or any of the other assorted cooking shows that populate (and are quite popular on) the Food Network and Travel Channel? If you have not, check them out. You will be amazed by the whirlwind of activity. Men and women chopping, dicing, slicing, muddling, stirring, whipping, pouring, measuring, and cooking up a whirling dervish in the kitchen. When they're done, what do you see? A happy chef, a smiling (and well-fed) host, and a plate of colorful, artfully prepared food worthy of a magazine cover.

What don't you see? Those men and women peeling the wrapping off a plastic container and tossing it in the microwave for 90 seconds before plopping down in front of the TV or computer with a glob of something that is barely recognizable as a food product on their plates.

My goal here isn't to turn you into a professional chef. Heck, I'm no professional chef. But I do want you to start embracing the active art of cooking with real food. I want you to engage in food preparation. I want you to be your own weight loss chef. That doesn't mean hours in the kitchen. I know we're all busy. But it does mean spending just a little more time to take care of yourself by taking care about the food that goes into your body. It means engaging your hands in the process of buying and making your food. It means engaging your brain in seeing what serving sizes should really look and feel like. It means serving yourself appropriate portions in an appropriate manner and on appropriate dinnerware. Because day in and day out and over the course of many months and years, the difference between a passive (e.g., microwaveable) meal and an active one can add up to many unwanted inches and pounds.

It's time to reverse that trend. During your time on the Active Calorie program, your goal is to make your eating more active. No need to do jumping jacks while you dine. This list of active-food purchasing, prepping, serving, and eating strategies—what I'm calling the Active Eating Habits—will make every meal a more deliberate, active process. You won't be able to do all of these every day. But do as many as you can as often as you can (or as often as makes sense)—at least one per day during the 4 weeks of the Active Calorie Diet. After a while, much of this should become automatic. Here's a look at the many ways you can activate your entire eating process, from food preparation to presentation and beyond.

Food Preparation

Preparing your own food is one of the key elements of Active Eating. I don't expect you to make everything from scratch, of course. But I do want you to go beyond the "open, nuke, and inhale" method of eating that so many of us call dinner (and often breakfast and lunch) these days. For one, making your own food burns twice as many calories as calling for delivery on your cell phone or sitting idly by for 5 minutes as a frozen dinner spins inside the microwave. By making your own food, you're also much more mindful of what kinds of foods you're putting in your mouth. You grow to appreciate food more and ultimately make better food choices and, yes, eat fewer calories and lose more weight. Here's how to activate your food selection and preparation. I've included in this list nearly every item I could think of. You certainly don't need them all. But read through and pick all of those that make sense for your food style and tastes.

Get (at least) one good knife: If you already have a set, great. If you don't, invest in at least one good kitchen knife. Trying to slice, dice, and chop vegetables with dull knives is a frustrating, if not mildly dangerous, exercise. With a good, sharp knife, you're much more likely to chop those fruits and veggies and carve freshly cooked meat because it's much easier. If you're going to buy more than one, I'd recommend a simple set of five or six knives that includes a chef's knife, a paring knife, a serrated knife, and a larger carving knife.

Go nonstick: I like a good nonstick pan for sautéing and baking. A well-seasoned cast-iron pan is also a good choice. Both allow you to avoid using gobs of butter or too much oil in favor of lighter, more flavorful options like wine, a mist of oil, vegetable stock, or fruit juice. Note: I have seen the research linking perfluoroalkyl acids like PFOA and PFOS, which give nonstick pans their heat resistance, to raised cholesterol levels in children. But that study was conducted on children who had been exposed to abnormally high levels after an industrial accident, not from eating scrambled eggs made on nonstick pans, which have considerably fewer levels of these chemicals.[1] The researchers themselves concluded that children's heart health was at a greater risk from what was going into those frying pans and from the children's increasing inactivity than from what the lining of the frying pan was made of.

Make lists: I never go to the grocery store without a list. Keep a running grocery list somewhere convenient in your kitchen. I recommend that about 80 percent of it (more if you can) come from the Active Calorie food categories.

Shop more often: The best way to keep an Active Calorie household is to shop a little more often. Instead of going to Costco and filling your freezer with army-size bags of hash browns and frozen burritos, go to a regular supermarket and buy a little less of fresh foods. It may increase your food bill a bit, but I promise you that you'll save money in health care costs down the road.

ACTIVE KITCHEN TOOLS AT A GLANCE

BEFORE YOU RUN OUT to the grocery store to stock up on Active Calorie foods, take a moment to survey your kitchen. You'll need a few supplies that will make Active Eating easier. You likely have many of them already; it's just a matter of pulling them out and making them more readily accessible. Here's all you need right now to activate your eating habits and start losing today.

- **CUTTING BOARDS**: You'll want a few of these for chopping fruits and veggies, slicing meats, and general food prep.

- **KNIVES**: See page 83. At least one good knife is a must.

- **MEASURING CUPS**: Dig them out and use them. You'll learn portions and drop pounds fast.

- **MEASURING SPOONS**: Same benefit as measuring cups.

- **UTENSILS**: Use them. Always.

- **SMALLER DISHWARE AND GLASSES**: These really do make a difference.

- **FOOD-STORAGE CONTAINERS**: Stash away the Couch Potato Calorie foods; display the Active Calorie foods.

Read the labels: Active-food selection means knowing what you're buying. You may think you do, but pick up that loaf of bread, flip it over, and read the label. Does it contain high fructose corn syrup? (It's surprising how many varieties do.) Then put it down and try another. Look for key Active Calorie ingredients, such as protein, fiber, and spices. Avoid Couch Potato Calorie ingredients, particularly lots of sugar, HFCS, trans fatty acids (hydrogenated oils), and low fiber.

Buy whole produce: You can buy nearly everything chopped and sliced and diced these days. That's okay when you're in a pinch. I'd absolutely rather have you eat prechopped veggies than none at all. But for the most part, I'd like you to buy whole fresh fruits and vegetables (you score bonus points if they're from a farmers' market) and clean and chop them instead of buying the prebagged kind. They taste better and often have more nutritional value.

Stock up on the spices: You're encouraged to use plenty of Active Calorie spices on this plan. Head to the spice and condiment sections of the store and stock up—many of them stay good for months or even years. Pick up pepper, garlic, low-sodium soy sauce, and vinegars of all kinds (my favorite is balsamic), as well as relishes, mustard, and salad dressings. When choosing ketchup, barbecue sauce, and other condiments, remember the previous advice: Read the labels. You'd be surprised by how many brands of ketchup use loads of HFCS.

Some of the test panelists noted that buying spices in little jars can get pricey. I recommend buying spices in bulk (they come in plastic bags instead of jars), which is far less expensive. Also, after the initial purchase, you won't have to spend money on spices again for a while. They last a long, long time. Whole spices (those not preground) can last up to 4 years in airtight containers stored in a cool, dry place. Strong spices like cinnamon, cloves, and pepper can last even longer. Ground spices have a shorter shelf life but will still be good for about 2 to 3 years if also stored in a cool, dry place in airtight containers. It's easy to tell if a spice is still good. Just give the container a shake, remove the cap, and have a sniff. If you can still smell the aroma of the spice, it's good to use. If there's no rich smell of spice, it's time to toss and replace it.

Measure it: We've reached a point in this country where our entire food supply has been supersized. Small ice cream cones have two, sometimes three, scoops; burgers weigh in at close to a pound; standard subs are a foot long—I could go on and on. But you get the idea. We need to get back to recognizing what healthy, appropriate portions look like. That's why I want you to dig out your measuring cups for 4 weeks and measure your portions. Use a 1- or 2-cup Pyrex measuring cup for fluids like 1% milk and a set of metal or plastic cups for solid measures like cooked pasta, rice, and whole grain cereal.

Weigh it: Many clients ask if they need a food scale. I used to say no, because I didn't want to take all the joy out of eating. But then I had a lightbulb moment when I realized that, used properly, a food scale can actually make eating pretty fun. How is that? Well, I talk a lot about proper portions, which are central to weight loss and maintenance. Most people have no clue what 4 ounces of meat or 1 ounce of cheese really looks like. So a food scale lets them see those sizes in no uncertain terms. Now, this may not be all that much fun in itself, but then my clients told me how they started playing around with their portions to make them feel bigger and more satisfying. Cherry Semple White, from the Active Calorie test panel, loves London broil. But she'd put a 3-ounce slab on the scale and feel sad about how little it looked. So she took to shaving it. "Suddenly I had a whole pile!" she said with glee. It took her longer to eat it; she got to savor the flavor; and she felt satisfied with a smaller, more appropriate portion. The same is true for cheese. I love cheese—love it. But 1 ounce doesn't go very far . . . unless you shred it. Then you can sprinkle it around and stretch it out over an entire meal. That's the positive power of a food scale.

Cook veggies crunchy: Raw veggies take the most energy to chew and digest. In fact, cooked carrots require 40 percent less energy to chew than uncooked ones. But there's a little trade-off with nutrition. Lightly cooking vegetables like carrots and broccoli helps break down their cells and makes the vitamins, minerals, and other plant nutrients more accessible. And let's face it: Many vegetables simply taste better cooked. The simple solution is to cook vegetables so that they're just tender enough to press through with a fork but still crisp and crunchy, not soft and mushy.

Order medium-rare: Naturally you're going to cook most of your meat through and through. But if you like your steak medium-rare to rare, you're in luck. Eating your meat on the rarer side of the doneness scale can boost the calories you burn digesting your meal by up to 12 percent. Note that ground meat is an exception to the rule. Cook and order it well done. It is a food-safety concern if underdone.

Serve up a salad: Filling half your plate with a fresh green salad is an excellent way to meet the Active Calorie Diet requirements. Yet so many of my clients rarely eat salad because it's a production to make. This is one case where I say go ahead and buy the bagged variety. You can get nearly any salad combination precleaned, cut, and ready to go. Or, even better, for about $25 you can get a Good Grips Salad Chopper and Bowl. I love this tool because it simplifies even the most complex salad. Simply throw all your ingredients—lettuce, veggies, fruits, and cheeses—into the bowl and glide the stainless steel blades through the mix. Voilà! Bite-size salad chunks in no time. Bonus: You can serve the salad right in the mixing bowl.

Spritz and spray: Olive oil and other healthy cooking fats are a welcome part of the Active Calorie Diet. But that doesn't mean I want you drowning your food in oil. Use one of the plastic spouts that allow you to drizzle small amounts of oil in your sautéing pan or on your salads. Or pick up a Misto Olive Oil Sprayer. This pump-action device sprays just enough oil to coat your cooking surface and foods.

Get steamed: Boiling vegetables can make them mushy and tasteless—plus you end up pouring too many vital nutrients, which are leeched into the water, straight down the drain. For a few bucks, you can buy a metal insert that turns any pot or saucepan into a steamer that's perfect for preparing broccoli, asparagus, beets, potatoes, corn, carrots, cauliflower, you name it! Steaming preserves the food's flavor and nutrients, but by themselves, steamed veggies can be kind of bland. Remember your warming Active Calories and liberally apply spices like garlic, ginger, balsamic vinegar, and freshly ground pepper.

Open the grill: Grilling is a very active way to prepare food that involves a lot of walking, flipping, basting, and general prep and care. Break free of the usual burgers and hot dogs and try grilling fish, lean cuts of pork, steak, vegetables, and even fruit! Grilled pineapple is divine. One smart Active Calorie cooking accessory to add to your grill: a grill basket. These hinged baskets are made with more tightly woven metal, so sliced zucchini and other smaller foods won't fall through the grill grate and into the fire. A basket also helps keep more fragile foods, like fish, from sticking to the grate or falling apart when you try to flip them.

Slow-cook it: No time to cook at the end of the day? Have it ready for you when you get home. Many of my clients find that a slow cooker makes homemade meals much easier. They simply toss their chicken and vegetables into the slow cooker in the morning and have a fabulous-smelling kitchen, with dinner ready to roll, when they walk through the door at the end of the day. Is it a necessity? No. Is it a nicety? You bet. Six quarts is a good size that will let you prepare family-size portions while you're at work.

Blend it: You might think that a blender is out of place in this batch, since the Active Calorie diet is all about chewing and eating whole foods. But it's also about filling up and feeling satisfied. There are many uses for a blender that will enable you to do just that. You can make delicious, fiber-filled, and very filling soup out of butternut squash. Some of my clients swear by a hand blender (Cuisinart makes a great one called the Smart Stick), which blends the ingredients right in whatever pot or bowl you're using. It saves lugging out a blender, and it requires much less cleanup.

Break away from baking: It's easy to get into a cooking rut. Many of us automatically set the oven to 350°F and toss in the chicken breasts without a second thought. As part of the Active Calorie Diet, I'd love for you to experiment with new cooking methods. Earlier, I mentioned grilling as a great Active Calorie cooking technique. But it's far from the only one. Roasting, stir-frying, and broiling are some of my other favorites. Roasting keeps vegetables firm but brings out the sweetness in root veggies like Brussels sprouts and parsnips. Stir-frying also uses a lot of veggies, keeps food firm, and often calls for a little heat, like chili oil, which is perfect for the Active Calorie Diet. A broiler pan will provide a quick and tasty alternative to baking for steaks, poultry, and especially fish, which is delicious broiled. Because it requires such high heat and cooks quickly, you also end up using less fat than you do with baking, which often involves fatty basting or, worse, breading.

Not sure how to get started? Consider taking a local cooking class with some gal pals. Test panelists Jeannette Johnson and Camilla Monti started their own. When they began following the Active Calorie Diet, they decided to get together to prepare meals each week; they called it

COT (Cook on Thursdays). Like exercising together, making meals is far more fun with a friend.

Think outside the breading box: Breading and bread crumbs are a way of life for some of my clients. They "shake and bake" chicken, eggplant, and pork chops and even toss bread crumbs into ground beef and turkey for burgers and meat loaves. I coax these clients away from commercial bread crumbs, which are generally doused in oil and even trans fats, and encourage them to substitute low-sugar, high-fiber crunchy breakfast cereals instead. Crushed Grape-Nuts or wheat flakes can provide a sweet coating and/or filling for many of your favorite dishes.

Add some zest: Pizzazz is the name of the game in the Active Calorie Diet. I love calorie-free add-ins that make your food pop with flavor without making you pop the buttons on your pants. Citrus zest—the colorful part of the rind of lemons, oranges, limes, etc.—is one of those. You can use a fine grater to add some zip to soups, salads, and grain dishes. If you find yourself zesting up all your favorite dishes, you can also get a Microplane Zester-Grater, which is perfectly graded to grate just the peel without digging into the white, bitter part of the rind. Sur La Table sells a superb one with an easy-to-hold gel-grip handle.

Peel it; press it: Many of my clients love fresh ginger but still let it shrivel and grow mold in the refrigerator because they don't like the hassle of peeling it with a paring knife. OXO Good Grips (a company known for making smart kitchen devices that feature ergonomic handles that anyone can grip and use) makes a ginger peeler that takes off the rough skin with an easily applied sharp blade while preserving the root. I'd add to this a Good Grips Garlic Press for the same reasons. Or try the Nextrend Garlic Twist Mincer. No more pounding and peeling stubborn cloves. This little gem crushes, peels, and minces garlic with a simple twist.

Grind it up: Nothing releases the flavor from chile peppers, garlic, or other dried spices like grinding. A good mortar and pestle (like the ones used to make fresh guacamole in Mexican restaurants) can take Active Calorie cooking to new heights! Along with delivering unsurpassable flavor, it's also really fun to use. You can get a small set for less than $10.

Or go whole hog and get a large stone set that pulls double duty as a stylish serving bowl.

Food Service

So many people plop their food—often a whole lot of food—onto their plates without thinking twice. The Active Calorie way is about mindful, not mindless, eating, and that includes how you serve yourself. *Mindless Eating* author Brian Wansink, PhD, has written a full volume (and then some) about the perils of automatic-pilot food consumption and how we have unwittingly piled on pounds by not paying attention to how much we're eating. Here's the Active Calorie solution for smarter, and ultimately slimmer, food service.

Rank your hunger: If we ate only when we were truly hungry, there'd be no overweight crisis in this country. I describe this in more detail on page 247, but I want you to create two mental scales. On the hunger scale, 1 is not hungry at all, while 5 is ravenous. On the fullness scale, 1 is still hungry, and 5 is stuffed to the gills. You want to move from a 3 on the hunger scale to a 3 on the fullness scale; right in the middle is where you'll feel energized and satisfied.

Measure out your portions: Just as I want you to get in the habit of measuring your food portions while you're cooking, do the same when you're serving. You'll find very specific serving sizes in the recipes. Take the time to break out the measuring cups and mete out the correct portions. It's important to learn what the appropriate amount of food looks like, especially since we've been supersized for the past decade and have truly lost touch with the amount of food we need to feel full.

Downsize your dishes (if yours are currently full size or larger): We eat with our eyes first, and everyone likes the look of a heaping plate. That's a problem when your plate is the size of a serving platter, as many are these days. Break out your salad dishes and shallow bowls. According to Dr. Wansink's research, when men and women eat off a plate that is just 2 inches smaller, they serve themselves 22 percent fewer calories per meal.[2] That's enough to drop 2 pounds in a month without doing anything else. Ditto for bowls, especially when you're serving up the sweet stuff. In one of his most frequently cited studies, Dr. Wansink invited 85 nutrition experts (read: people who should really know better) to an ice cream social. The foodies got either a 17- or 34-ounce bowl, along with a 2- or 3-ounce ice cream scoop to serve themselves. Not surprisingly, the folks with the big bowls and scoops ate more. What is surprising is how much more. Those who received the large bowls ate 31 percent more ice cream—about 130 calories' worth. Those who had both large bowls and scoops dished out 57 percent more—that's an additional 200 calories' worth—than those who had small bowls and scoops.[3]

Watch your glasses, too. The same optical illusions apply. Research at Dr. Wansink's Food and Brand Lab at the University of Illinois at Urbana-Champaign found that when people poured themselves beverages in short, wide glasses, they ended up with 76 percent more soda, juice, or milk than when they used tall, slender glassware.[4]

Camilla Monti from the test panel took this advice to the next level by purchasing "portion" plates online. These pretty plates are painted with guidelines for how much of each type of food should go where (much like the graphic on page 11). Though the portions don't directly correlate with the Active Calorie guidelines, they're pretty close (especially with starchy carbs and proteins) and can be a great weight loss tool. The Diet Plate and the Balance Plate are two popular brands.

Serve yourself restaurant style: Having soup and/or salad along with your main meal? Serve it one course at a time, the way they do in restaurants, rather than all at once. When you feed yourself in courses, you'll eat more slowly, feel full sooner, think about how much more food you really need, and be less inclined to take seconds. Have your salad or soup first. Take your time, and think about how hungry you still are before serving yourself the main course.

Serve from the stove: Your serving platters may be pretty, but placing all the food you just prepared on the table for an eating free-for-all ramps up the potential for eating more than you need or even want,

(continued on page 94)

{ camilla monti }

She Made It Her Own

AGE: 60
POUNDS LOST:
8.6
INCHES LOST:
7 including 2½ off her waist

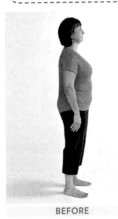

BEFORE

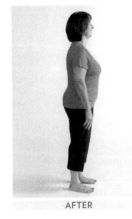

AFTER

THE GOAL of the Active Calorie Diet is to set you on a path you can stay on for the rest of your life. That path is going to be slightly different for everyone. Some people will follow the recipes to the letter and make many of these dishes a permanent part of their lives. Others may never make a single recipe, but they'll walk away with the spirit of the eating plan. And some, like Camilla Monti, will take the plan and make it their own.

"I'm a big foodie. I love to cook. I always have. But this plan has been amazing for helping me see outside my box and imagine new food combinations and new ways to season and spice things. I've adopted so many things that I would never have thought of before," she told me with great enthusiasm at our 4-week check-in. "You know you get into a rut with the foods you eat, always making the same dishes and using the same flavorings without even meaning to. This diet changed all that for me. Now I'm putting cayenne pepper in my pomegranate tea! I'm making mint chutney. I'm seeing food in a whole new way. I don't need all the bread. I can have tuna and beans on Wasa Crisps. I don't have to drink plain water. I can have these great teas. I'm breaking up and baking pita bread instead of eating nacho chips. There's so much possibility. I'm more excited about going forward than I was about getting started!"

A social creature by nature, Camilla is also thrilled that she can continue her girls' nights out and dinners at restaurants in town without sacrificing her weight loss

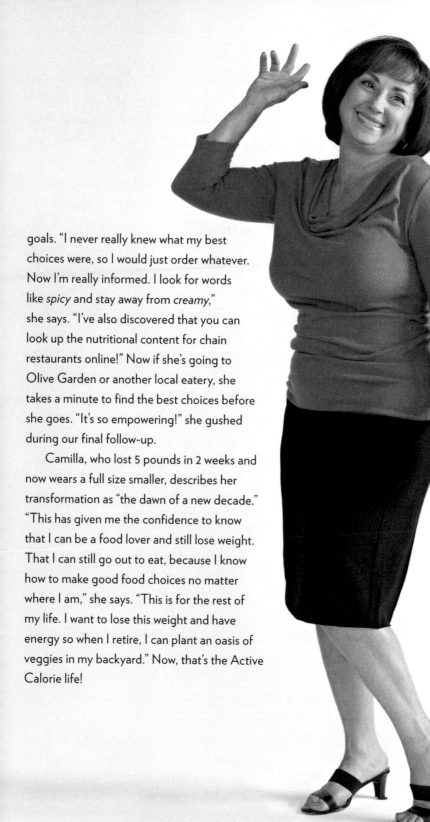

goals. "I never really knew what my best choices were, so I would just order whatever. Now I'm really informed. I look for words like *spicy* and stay away from *creamy*," she says. "I've also discovered that you can look up the nutritional content for chain restaurants online!" Now if she's going to Olive Garden or another local eatery, she takes a minute to find the best choices before she goes. "It's so empowering!" she gushed during our final follow-up.

Camilla, who lost 5 pounds in 2 weeks and now wears a full size smaller, describes her transformation as "the dawn of a new decade." "This has given me the confidence to know that I can be a food lover and still lose weight. That I can still go out to eat, because I know how to make good food choices no matter where I am," she says. "This is for the rest of my life. I want to lose this weight and have energy so when I retire, I can plant an oasis of veggies in my backyard." Now, that's the Active Calorie life!

because everyone keeps picking long past the point of hunger until all the food is gone. Instead, keep the food in the pots and pans on the stove and make your plates from there. When you're done, put the food away. A new Cornell study found that people ate up to 35 percent less food when they used this food-service strategy.[5]

Table it: Even if you're eating alone, put your food on a plate, take it out of the kitchen, and sit down to a nice meal at a table, where you can relax and unwind from the day. This is especially important if you live alone, in fact. Too often, my clients barely remember eating because they simply stand in front of the refrigerator or hunker over the sink spooning food from a plastic container directly into their mouths. It may seem paradoxical, but Active Eating in this case involves sitting down. That means snacks, too.

Use your utensils: Even if you're eating a sandwich or a burger, take the time to get out a fork and knife and cut it in half. Cut all food into small pieces. Put down your fork between each bite as you chew. These are habits that will let you enjoy your food to the fullest without feeling the urge to overeat. One of my favorite tricks when I'm eating Asian food like sushi is to use chopsticks. It really slows you down and makes you mindful of every bite.

Take smaller bites and chew more: Take the same-size bite you normally do and cut it in half (most of us gulp our food without even thinking about it). Then chew it 10 to 12 times. I know you've probably heard that you should chew your food 30 times. Frankly, that's unreasonable. But many of us take a few chomps and swallow food partially whole.

Give thanks. Saying grace has always been a beautiful ritual of being thankful for your food before you eat it. It doesn't matter what religion you are or, frankly, even if you have a religion. It's about appreciating the food in front of you and being grateful for having it, something that has been largely lost in our all-you-can-eat culture. But if you take a moment before you start eating to look at the food in front of you, appreciate the food in front of you, and give thanks for the food in front of you, I promise that you will be far less likely to mindlessly pig out.

Food Storage

Where do you keep your food? In clear containers? Stashed in the pantry? Are the cookies on the countertop? How about those vegetables? Most of us don't give too much thought to where we store our food. We just put it away. It's time to activate your food storage, too. Research shows that where you keep your food can have a big impact on what and how much you eat. Here's the Active Calorie way.

Clean the cupboards: Clutter is bad for healthy decision making. Clean house and purge your kitchen and pantry of those stale marshmallows, old bags of chips, long-unfinished cereal boxes, and other foods that are just taking up space and may be tempting you to eat easily accessible junk that you really don't want but will reach for in moments of weakness simply because it's convenient. Once the real junk is out of the way, go back through with a scrupulous Active Calorie eye. Read your labels and toss out foods that have Couch Potato Calorie sources as their top ingredients. That means ditching foods rich in HFCS, refined flour, hydrogenated oils (trans fats), and sugar. Feeling guilty about throwing away food? Don't. Remember that there are two ways to waste food: in the trash and around your own waist. Carrying around excess pounds isn't going to help starving people in any country. Besides, junk is junk. The processed, nutrient-barren food you're throwing out wouldn't provide much nourishment to those who truly need it most.

Put treats out of sight: You can have sweets and chips in the house (within reason; remember, if it's there, you'll eat it). But stash them on the highest shelves you have, preferably hidden from view. It seems like a small step, but it makes you stop and think and actively seek out your treat—which you will do when you really want it. And when you are actually just bored, you won't. Studies have shown that men and women eat far fewer sweets that are stored in opaque containers, obscuring what's inside, rather than clear jars. In fact, in one study from the University of Illinois, researchers found that office workers ate 25 percent fewer Hershey's Kisses when they were placed inside a

AVOID MINDLESS MUNCHING

COOKING MORE IS PART OF the Active Calorie life. But there's a hidden peril that I would be remiss if I didn't address—tasting and picking and accumulating lots of mindless calories in the process. Though you'll be munching on healthier fare than if you ordered out, all those little nibbles you take while you prepare your meals can add up quickly—I've seen women take in 500 calories before they even put their food on a plate.

Similarly, postmeal, there's nearly unconscious grazing when everyone picks at the leftovers long past the point of hunger. Serving from the stove will reduce this temptation, but if you're the guest at a party where all the food is spread out in front of you, here are some strategies that can help.

- **CHEW GUM.** This will keep your mouth busy and burn a few extra calories, plus the minty fresh taste won't mix well with most foods.

- **BRUSH UP.** Head to the bathroom and brush your teeth after eating. The mint flavor will reduce the urge to nibble, as will your freshly cleaned teeth and gums.

- **LEAVE THE EVIDENCE.** When eating or drinking in an "all you can chow down" environment like a buffet or wedding, try to hold onto some evidence of your consumption. Hang onto the cocktail napkins that come with your appetizers and drinks as visual reminders of how many you've had.

slightly inconvenient spot out of sight, such as inside a desk drawer, than when they were within arm's reach in plain view.[6]

Play up that produce: So if you put the Couch Potato Calories out of sight, where do you think you should you put your Active Calories? Exactly: in plain view. Wash, slice, and arrange fresh fruits and veggies in clear bowls and plastic bags on easy-to-reach, eye-level spots in the fridge. Do the same in the pantry. Put nuts and beef jerky, roasted soybeans, and other Active Calorie snacks on the easy-to-access shelves.

Label your spices: If you're like me, your spice cabinet overfloweth with spices you bought for a special recipe and never cracked open again. Rifle through there and find the ones that serve as warming

Active Calories. Take a marker and write "Warm" on the ones that fit the bill, and place them front and center on the shelves.

Create your own grab-and-gos: Instead of buying individually packaged snack packs and frozen-food meals, create your own for Active Calorie convenience. Small, reusable storage containers are ideal for nuts, popcorn, baby carrots, grapes, grape tomatoes, and other grab-and-go foods. Likewise, prepare some of the recipes you'll find in Chapter 7, divide them into appropriate portions in zip-top bags or plastic containers, and freeze them for later.

Pack it: Yes, it's more work. But packing your lunch and snacks not only saves you money but also spares fat—around your waist. For added incentive, take the $10 you would spend on lunch and snacks every day and put it in a jar. Treat yourself to a trip at the end of the year with the several grand you'll have saved.

Food Environment

People eat more in noisy, bustling environments than they do in ones that are more serene. We also eat more when we're distracted. The ambience that surrounds your eating experience influences what and how much you eat more than you think. Here's how to set the best stage for Active Eating.

Turn off the television: When you go to Italy or another European country, food is the main event. People there spend hours lingering over each dish, having conversations, and appreciating their food. In our always-on-the-go society in this country, food is all too often an afterthought, if a thought at all. Eating is something we do while we're doing something else, like watching TV. Research shows that people who nosh while they watch TV eat more food and more often, enough to add up to an extra meal each day. Get off the sofa, turn off the TV, sit down at a table, and enjoy your meal and the company of family or friends.

Shed light on your meals: There's a reason restaurants dim the lights: so you'll eat more. Whether it's because darkness sends us into hibernation mode or simply lowers our inhibitions, we toss back more calories in dimly lit environments. Open the curtains, buy some higher-wattage bulbs, and let the bright light shine in your kitchen and dining room. Sunny, well-lit spaces also lift your mood, which makes you less likely to overeat.

Mirror, mirror on the wall . . . People who are unhappy with their weight tend to avoid mirrors. I encourage you to hang a few in the places you need them most: the dining room and kitchen. Do I want to torture you? No. Do I want you to stay mindful of your mission to make a healthy lifestyle change? Yes. The mirrors not only serve as reflective strings around your finger but also brighten up the room (see previous tip) and will keep you moving. You're less likely to slump over the kitchen counter with a pint of mint chocolate chip ice cream or mindlessly spoon serving after serving of holiday stuffing onto your plate when you can catch glimpses of yourself in action. What you will do is sit up straight, think about what you're doing, eat a little less, smile a little more, and keep moving.

Clear the clutter: Okay, be honest. Step into your kitchen. Can you find the counter? If there's a table in there, can you see slivers of wood peeking through all the bills, magazines, stacks of unread junk mail, reports from your kids' schools, and other bric-a-brac that was tossed atop of it and has yet to be tended to? Kitchens and kitchen tables are some of the greatest repositories for the clutter of our lives. But let's face it: No one wants to eat among that chaos. It's stressful (which makes you eat more) at best, impossible at worst (and you're back to leaning over the sink with a sandwich in hand). You're also far less likely to cook in the first place if the kitchen resembles tornado wreckage. Take an hour before starting the Active Calorie plan and clear the clutter. Find a pretty basket for the bills and loose papers, and declare the kitchen a no-dumping zone.

Journal it: Last but far from least, keep a journal in the kitchen and jot down what you're eating, how much, and the mood you're in. A simple journal is the most powerful weight loss tool available. I've provided some pages at the end of this book to get you started; you can either copy these pages to use through the 4-week plan or visit www. prevention.com/shop (or call 800-848-4735) to get your *Active Calorie Diet Journal*. And don't stop after those 4 weeks. Continue until you reach your weight loss goal. We eat for so many reasons that have nothing to do with filling our bellies. One national survey by the Calorie Control Council found that 36 percent of women often eat for emotional reasons (fewer men do this, but they're not immune).[7] By journaling, you will learn a lot not only about what but also, more important, why you eat. Those lessons will help you keep off the weight once it's gone.

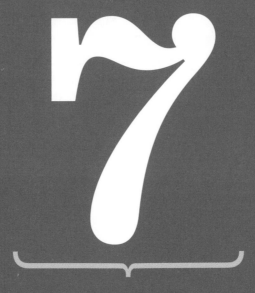

Cook More:
Active Calorie Recipes

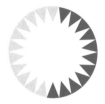

Before they started the plan, more than a few of the Active Calorie Diet test panelists were skeptical. "I don't usually eat protein in the morning." "I don't like spice." "I'm not much of a vegetable person." You could feel the apprehension nearly oozing out of their pores as they spoke, flipping through the menus. But in just 4 weeks' time, they were glowing (in some cases literally, with clearer, brighter skin) with enthusiasm about how much they loved the food. "I would never have thought of that!" "Who knew I liked _____?!" "I'm looking at food in a whole new way!" Even those who didn't follow the recipes to the letter were thrilled at how the Active Calorie Diet opened their minds to new food combinations.

Little wonder, really. A recent survey of 4,000 families revealed that most women rely on just nine different meals—spaghetti, pizza, and casseroles being among them—that they put into heavy rotation to feed themselves and their families. (Only women were surveyed, but my experience is that men fall into the same food ruts.) One in four women even has set days for which she makes each dish. That's why healthy cooking can be so challenging for so many people. When they leave their comfort zones, they feel confused. "Every time I've lost weight before, it was the 'bland food' diet," says test panelist Melissa

{ melissa schilling }

A Journey of Discovery

AGE: 45
POUNDS LOST:
5
INCHES LOST:
3

MELISSA SCHILLING is no stranger to dieting. What was far less familiar to her was flavor and fullness. "I've never been a big vegetable person. So when I wanted to lose weight, it was the same thing—chicken and brown rice in the slow-cooker," she recalls. "Who knew I liked mango? Who knew I loved edamame? I'd never even heard of edamame!"

She was also delighted by how filling she found the food. "The breakfast parfait was the best! I loved it. So big and so filling," she says. "I also love the flexibility of the plan. If I didn't like one thing, I could find another that I really liked. I started experimenting with making my own spicy sandwich spreads, like putting cracked pepper in light mayo."

The result is a way of eating that she's hooked on for life. "It's as easy as changing the emphasis of what you put on your plate," she says. "I can do that for every meal while still having filling, delicious food. It's a little more work to think ahead and pack my lunch. But the weight loss and endless energy are worth it."

Schilling, 45. "It was always chicken and turkey and brown rice. You get bored pretty quickly." She and the others were anything but bored on the Active Calorie Diet.

By using so many warming spices—like ginger, cloves, and cinnamon—as well as chile peppers in unusual ways, you can make even old standbys like chicken and fish taste exciting and new. Speaking of warming spices and peppers, many of the panelists were pleasantly surprised at how full these foods made them feel. "This is the first diet I've ever done that I'm not hungry on!" Jackie Detty, 34, who lost 4.6 pounds and 7½ inches in 4 weeks, told me. "The initial prep took some time, but it was worth it. Now it's easy to follow." Kathy Schmidt, 59, who lost 7.8 pounds and 9 inches during the program, told me that this diet had the most positive effects of any she'd ever been on (and there have been a few). "I'm shocked how quickly I feel full," she says, crediting the increased heat and protein with leaving her satisfied rather than starving as she shed pounds. All of the test panelists plan to continue eating the Active Calorie way.

Now it's your turn to break out of your bland "diet"-food box and have your own Active Calorie awakening. In the pages that follow, you'll find almost 80 recipes for breakfast, lunch, dinner, and snacks and desserts. Each recipe gives you a complete Active Calorie meal and follows the meal-composition guidelines in Chapter 5. You'll see that the breakdown of carbs to proteins to fats doesn't always match the 50-25-25 percentage exactly; nor are the calorie counts or grams of fiber exactly what's called for in the meal composition (especially in the snacks and desserts). That's okay. Again, I don't want you to go crazy counting calories or calculating the nutritional ratios. The meal-composition guidelines are just that—guidelines to give you an approximation of the nutrition you need. Feel free to skip over the guidelines and the nutritional analysis completely, if you want; we've done the work for you!

So all you need to do is pick and choose, mix and match, to your heart's content for the next 4 weeks. By the end of the month, you'll be lighter and more energetic and have a whole new assortment of delicious foods in your repertoire. Turn the page and let's get cooking.

Breakfast

I know it will be an adjustment for many of you to eat breakfast at all, much less a substantial breakfast, but it really helps set the stage for an active day. All of the following recipes provide around 400 calories from chewy proteins and hearty fiber-rich foods; they are also quick and easy to make.

COOKIE-CRUNCH SMOOTHIE

Prep time: 5 minutes / Total time: 10 minutes / Serves 1 (2 cups per serving)

³⁄₄	cup fat-free milk
1	banana
4	ice cubes
3	chocolate cookie wafers
2¹⁄₂	tablespoons ground flaxseed
2	teaspoons sugar
¹⁄₂	teaspoon vanilla extract

Place the milk, banana, ice cubes, chocolate wafers, flaxseed, sugar, and vanilla extract in a blender. Blend until smooth and serve immediately.

PER SERVING: 398 calories, 12 g protein, 64 g carbohydrates, 9 g fiber, 11 g fat (1 g saturated), 222 mg sodium

PEANUT BUTTER SMOOTHIE

Prep time: 5 minutes / Total time: 5 minutes / Serves 1 (2¼ cups per serving)

½	cup 0% fat plain Greek yogurt
¾	cup fat-free milk
½	banana
½	cup high-fiber cereal flakes
1	tablespoon ground flaxseed
1	tablespoon peanut butter
1	tablespoon bittersweet chocolate chips
2	teaspoons packed light brown sugar
½	teaspoon vanilla extract
2	ice cubes

Place the yogurt, milk, banana, cereal, flaxseed, peanut butter, chocolate chips, brown sugar, vanilla extract, and ice cubes in a blender. Blend until smooth. Serve immediately.

PER SERVING: 405 calories, 21 g protein, 61g carbohydrates, 7 g fiber, 9 g fat (3 g saturated), 272 mg sodium

CHEF'S NOTE: If you have bananas that are starting to become overripe, toss them in the freezer and use them in smoothies like this one.

PUMPKIN-MAPLE OATMEAL

Prep time: 2 minutes / Total time: 10 minutes / Serves 1 (1³⁄₄ cups per serving)

1 cup fat-free milk

¹⁄₂ cup old-fashioned oats

1 teaspoon grated fresh ginger

¹⁄₂ teaspoon ground cinnamon

1 apple, cubed

1 tablespoon canned pumpkin

1 tablespoon chopped pecans

1 teaspoon maple syrup

1. Place the milk, oats, ginger, cinnamon, and apple in a small saucepan. Bring to a boil, then reduce to a simmer. Cook for 5 minutes, or until most of the liquid is absorbed.

2. Swirl in the pumpkin and sprinkle with pecans. Drizzle with maple syrup and serve immediately.

PER SERVING: 418 calories, 16 g protein, 71 g carbohydrates, 10 g fiber, 8 g fat (0 g saturated), 130 mg sodium

CHEF'S NOTE: You can substitute walnuts or hazelnuts for the pecans, if you prefer.

STRAWBERRIES-AND-CREAM HOT CEREAL

**Prep time: 5 minutes / Total time: 10 minutes /
Serves 1 (1$^1/_2$ cups cereal with topping per serving)**

1$^1/_2$ cups fat-free milk

$^1/_3$ cup dry toasted wheat cereal, such as Wheatena

3 tablespoons part-skim ricotta cheese

2 teaspoons powdered sugar

$^1/_4$ teaspoon vanilla extract

$^1/_2$ cup chopped fresh strawberries (about 3 large strawberries)

1. Place the milk in a small saucepan over medium heat. When the milk begins to simmer, stir in the cereal. Reduce the heat to low and cook for 4 to 5 minutes, stirring often.

2. Place the cheese in a small bowl, along with the sugar and vanilla extract. Stir until well combined.

3. Transfer the cereal to a small bowl and top with the cheese. Scatter the chopped strawberries over the cheese and serve immediately.

PER SERVING: 412 calories, 24 g protein, 67 g carbohydrates, 7 g fiber, 5 g fat (2 g saturated), 219 mg sodium

CHEF'S NOTE: This can be made with any berry, such as blueberries, cherries, or raspberries.

RASPBERRY-ALMOND BREAKFAST PARFAIT

Prep time: 5 minutes / Total time: 5 minutes / Serves 1 (1½ cups per serving)

8	ounces (1 cup) 0% fat plain Greek yogurt
½	cup raspberries
2	tablespoons almonds, chopped
¼	teaspoon almond extract
½	teaspoon ground cinnamon
	Pinch of cayenne
¾	cup high-fiber cereal

1. Place the yogurt, ¼ cup of the raspberries, the almonds, almond extract, cinnamon, and cayenne in a small bowl. Mash with a spoon until the berries break apart and all the ingredients are well combined.

2. Sprinkle half the cereal into the bottom of a glass parfait dish or bowl. Top with the yogurt mixture, then sprinkle with the remaining cereal and ¼ cup berries. Serve immediately or store in the fridge for up to 1 day.

PER SERVING: 372 calories, 27 g protein, 43 g carbohydrates, 10 g fiber, 10 g fat (0 g saturated), 282 mg sodium

CHEF'S NOTE: Don't be afraid to use the cayenne; it won't make the parfait spicy but will add just a hint of warmth to the raspberries.

You can substitute a regular low-fat plain yogurt for the Greek yogurt, if you prefer, but it will make your parfait thinner. If you chill the parfait before eating, the yogurt will thicken and the cereal will soften.

You can also enjoy with hot or iced unsweetened green tea.

FRENCH SCRAMBLED EGGS

Prep time: 10 minutes / Total time: 15 minutes /
Serves 4 (about 1 cup scrambled eggs with topping and 2 ounces baguette per serving)

4	egg whites
2	eggs
$\frac{1}{2}$	cup 0% fat plain Greek yogurt
2	tablespoons chopped parsley
2	tablespoons chopped chives
2	tablespoons chopped tarragon or basil
8	ounces frozen artichokes, thawed and chopped
4	ounces Brie cheese, thinly sliced
8	ounces whole wheat baguette, toasted

1. Place the egg whites, eggs, yogurt, parsley, chives, and tarragon or basil in a medium bowl. Whisk to combine.

2. Heat a large skillet over medium heat. Coat with cooking spray and add the egg mixture. Cook for 2 to 3 minutes, stirring once or twice, or until the eggs are almost cooked through.

3. Scatter the artichokes and cheese over the top. Cover and cook for 1 minute, or until the cheese is melted. Serve immediately with the baguette.

PER SERVING: 379 calories, 25 g protein, 45 g carbohydrates, 5 g fiber, 13 g fat (6 g saturated), 756 mg sodium

CHEF'S NOTE: If you don't like Brie, try goat cheese, which is lower in fat.

EGGS AND TOMATOES

Prep time: 5 minutes / Total time: 10 minutes /
Serves 4 (2 eggs plus $\frac{1}{2}$ cup topping and 1 slice bread per serving)

1	teaspoon olive oil
1	small red onion, chopped
1	green bell pepper, seeded and chopped
	Pinch of red-pepper flakes
1	cup jarred marinara sauce
8	eggs
$\frac{1}{3}$	cup shredded part-skim mozzarella cheese
$\frac{1}{4}$	cup chopped basil
8	ounces crusty country-style whole wheat bread, sliced into 4 pieces, toasted

1. Heat a large skillet over medium heat. Coat with cooking spray and add the oil. Add the onion and bell pepper and cook for 4 to 5 minutes, stirring often, or until the onion and bell pepper start to brown.

2. Add the red-pepper flakes and cook for 1 minute longer.

3. Reduce the heat to low and arrange the onion and bell pepper around the edges of the skillet. Carefully pour the marinara sauce in the center of the skillet and crack the eggs over the sauce. Sprinkle the cheese over the eggs. Cover and cook for 2 to 3 minutes, or until the whites are firm and the yolks start to cook around the edges.

4. Sprinkle with the basil and immediately serve the eggs with the sauce, onion, and bell pepper on top of the toast.

PER SERVING: 376 calories, 21 g protein, 43 g carbohydrates, 3 g fiber, 12 g fat (4 g saturated), 714 mg sodium

BACON-AND-BROCCOLI EGG SANDWICH

Prep time: 5 minutes / Total time: 10 minutes /
Serves 1 (1 sandwich and 1 small apple or pear per serving)

1	egg
1	egg white
1	teaspoon hot sauce
½	cup broccoli florets, roughly chopped
2	slices nitrate-free turkey bacon, chopped
½	ounce part-skim mozzarella cheese (about 2 tablespoons)
2	slices high-fiber whole grain bread
1	romaine lettuce leaf, cut in half
1	small apple or pear

1. Place the egg, egg white, and hot sauce in a small bowl. Whisk to combine.

2. Heat a small skillet over high heat. Coat with cooking spray and add the broccoli and bacon. Stir once and reduce the heat to low. Cover and cook for 1 to 2 minutes, stirring once or twice, or until the broccoli is tender-crisp.

3. Increase the heat to medium and add the egg and cheese. Cover and cook for another 2 minutes, stirring once, or until the egg is cooked through.

4. Toast the bread. Transfer the eggs to the bun and top with the lettuce. Serve immediately or wrap in aluminum foil. Have 1 small apple or pear on the side.

PER SERVING: 407 calories, 35 g protein, 46 g carbohydrates, 11 g fiber, 12 g fat (3 g saturated), 550 mg sodium

CHEF'S NOTE: You can substitute any type of lettuce other than iceberg for the romaine. Darker lettuces like romaine have a higher nutritional value than light ones like iceberg.

BIRDIES IN A BASKET

Prep time: 5 minutes / Total time: 10 minutes /
Serves 1 (2 slices toast and 1 cup filling per serving)

2	slices whole wheat toast with a 2"-diameter circle cut out from the center
2	eggs
$\frac{1}{4}$	teaspoon freshly ground black pepper
$\frac{1}{8}$	teaspoon cayenne
1	cup canned artichokes, rinsed and drained
1	tomato, sliced

1. Heat a large skillet over medium heat. Coat with cooking spray. Add the bread slices toward the center of the skillet and place the circles around the edges.

2. Crack an egg into each bread hole, sprinkle with the pepper and cayenne, and cook for 3 minutes, or until the white of each egg is no longer translucent. Spray the surface of the egg-filled bread with another thin layer of cooking spray.

3. Carefully flip the bread and top with the artichokes and tomato slices. Cook for 1 to 2 minutes longer, or until the white of each egg is cooked when pierced with a knife. Serve immediately.

PER SERVING: 413 calories, 25 g protein, 46 g carbohydrates, 18 g fiber, 14 g fat (3 g saturated), 484 mg

SOUTHWESTERN BREAKFAST BURRITO

Prep time: 5 minutes / Total time: 10 minutes /
Serves 4 (one 10" tortilla with 1¼ cups filling per serving)

4 high-fiber whole grain sandwich wraps (10" diameter)

4 egg whites

2 eggs

1 cup no-salt-added canned black beans, rinsed and drained

½ green bell pepper, finely chopped

½ red bell pepper, finely chopped

½ small red onion, finely chopped

2 tablespoons pickled jalapeño chile pepper rings, chopped

1 cup shredded reduced-fat Cheddar cheese

3 tablespoons jarred spicy salsa

1. Wrap the sandwich wraps in aluminum foil and cook for 5 to 7 minutes in a toaster oven on medium or in an oven preheated to 350°F.

2. Place the egg whites, eggs, and beans in a medium bowl and whisk until just combined.

3. Heat a larger skillet over medium heat for 30 seconds. Coat with cooking spray. Add the egg mixture. Cook for 1 minute, or until the edges are no longer translucent, then stir with a spatula.

4. Sprinkle the top of the eggs with the green and red bell peppers, onion, chile pepper rings, and cheese. Reduce the heat to low and cover. Cook for 1 minute longer, or until the eggs are cooked through and the cheese is melted.

5. Set out the sandwich wraps. Place a quarter of the mixture on each wrap, and divide the salsa among the wraps evenly. Fold in the 2 sides of each wrap to close. Wrap in aluminum foil or serve immediately.

PER SERVING: 383 calories, 23 g protein, 44 g carbohydrates, 11 g fiber, 13 g fat (3 g saturated), 717 mg sodium

HAM-AND-CHEESE BAKE

Prep time: 10 minutes / Total time: 40 minutes /
Serves 4 (1½ cups casserole with one 8-ounce glass orange or
grapefruit juice per serving)

½	cup fat-free milk
½	cup 0% fat plain Greek yogurt
4	eggs
4	egg whites
3	tablespoons ground flaxseed
1	teaspoon dried oregano
4	ounces whole wheat bread, cubed
2	cups broccoli florets, chopped
2	scallions or 1 shallot, chopped
2	slices Canadian bacon or ham, chopped (about 1½ ounces)
2	tomatoes, sliced
½	cup (about 4 ounces) crumbled feta cheese
8	ounces orange or grapefruit juice

1. Preheat the oven to 350°F. Place the milk, yogurt, eggs, egg whites, flaxseed, and oregano in a large bowl. Whisk until well combined.

2. Add the bread, broccoli, scallions or shallot, and bacon or ham and stir until the mixture is well coated. Transfer to an 8" × 8" baking dish.

3. Top with the tomatoes and sprinkle with the cheese. Bake for 20 to 25 minutes, or until the cheese is slightly browned and the top of the casserole puffs. Cut into 4 equal portions and serve immediately with 1 glass of orange or grapefruit juice.

PER SERVING: 373 calories, 23 g protein, 48 g carbohydrates, 4 g fiber, 10 g fat (4 g saturated), 652 mg sodium

STUFFED BLUEBERRY FRENCH TOAST

Prep time: 10 minutes / Total time: 20 minutes /
Serves 4 (2 slices bread with $1/2$ cup filling per serving)

2	cups blueberries
1	cup fat-free milk
$1/2$	cup 1% cottage cheese
$1/3$	cup sugar
2	large egg whites
1	large egg
1	teaspoon vanilla extract
8	slices firm country-style whole wheat bread
1	tablespoon canola oil

1. Place the blueberries, $1/2$ cup of the milk, the cottage cheese, and sugar in a blender or food processor. Blend until smooth.

2. Place the egg whites, egg, vanilla extract, and remaining $1/2$ cup milk in a shallow bowl and whisk until smooth.

3. Divide the blueberry mixture among 4 of the slices of bread and top with the remaining 4 bread slices.

4. Heat a large skillet over medium heat. Add $1/2$ tablespoon of the oil and place the stuffed bread into the skillet. Cook for 2 to 3 minutes, or until the bread starts to brown.

5. Drizzle the remaining oil over the top of the bread and turn. Cook for 2 to 3 minutes longer, or until browned and cooked through. Serve immediately or cool on a wire rack.

PER SERVING: 389 calories, 17 g protein, 64 g carbohydrates, 7 g fiber, 7 g fat (0 g saturated), 456 mg sodium

CHEF'S NOTE: This stuffed toast is delicious cold the next day and can be wrapped in aluminum foil to take on the road.

BUCKWHEAT PANCAKES WITH SMOKED SALMON

Prep time: 20 minutes / Total time: 30 minutes /
Serves 4 (2 pancakes with 1 ounce smoked salmon and ¼ cup cucumbers
with sour cream per serving)

1	small cucumber, thinly sliced
¼	small red onion or small shallot, minced
¼	cup reduced-fat sour cream
1	tablespoon fresh lemon juice
1	tablespoon chopped fresh dill or chives
⅛	teaspoon cayenne
1½	cups buckwheat pancake mix
1	teaspoon sugar
1	cup fat-free milk
3	egg whites
1	tablespoon canola oil
4	ounces thinly sliced smoked salmon, cut into small pieces

1. Place the cucumber, onion or shallot, sour cream, lemon juice, dill or chives, and cayenne in a medium bowl. Toss to coat. Set aside.

2. Place the pancake mix and sugar in a large bowl. Whisk to combine. Add the milk, egg whites, and oil. Stir until no lumps remain.

3. Heat a griddle or large skillet over high heat. Coat with a light layer of cooking spray. Spoon out ¼ cup of the batter, leaving 1" between each dollop. Cook for 2 to 3 minutes, or until small bubbles form on the top of each pancake and the edges are dry. Flip and repeat.

4. Transfer the pancakes to a platter and top with the smoked salmon and cucumber mixture.

PER SERVING: 405 calories, 31 g protein, 42 g carbohydrates, 8 g fiber, 10 g fat (2 g saturated), 433 mg sodium

CHEF'S NOTE: You can swap whole wheat or whole grain pancake mix for the buckwheat, if you prefer.

BLUEBERRY-WALNUT PANCAKES WITH CARDAMOM

Prep time: 5 minutes / Total time: 20 minutes /
Serves 4 (three 5″ pancakes with 1 tablespoon syrup per serving)

2	cups whole wheat or whole grain pancake mix
3	tablespoons ground golden flaxseed
1	teaspoon ground cardamom or cinnamon
1¼	cups fresh blueberries
⅓	cup toasted walnuts, chopped
1¼	cups fat-free milk
3	egg whites
¼	cup water
¼	cup pure maple syrup

1. Place the pancake mix, flaxseed, and cardamom or cinnamon in a large bowl. Mix until combined.

2. Make a well in the center of the pancake mix and add the blueberries, walnuts, milk, egg whites, and water. Working from the center of the wet ingredients, stir about 15 turns with a wooden spoon, or until the pancake mix is just combined.

3. Heat a griddle over high heat. Coat with cooking spray. Scoop ⅓ cup of the batter and place on the griddle, spacing the pancakes 1″ apart. Cook for 2 to 3 minutes, or until bubbles form around the edges. Turn and cook for 2 to 3 minutes longer, or until the pancakes are cooked through.

4. Repeat with the remaining pancake batter. Transfer the pancakes to a large serving platter and drizzle with the syrup. Serve immediately.

PER SERVING: 397 calories, 14 g protein, 66 g carbohydrates, 8 g fiber, 11 g fat (1 g saturated), 517 mg sodium

ALMOND-PEAR WAFFLES

Prep time: 5 minutes / Total time: 30 minutes / Serves 5 (one 8″ waffle per serving)

2	cups multigrain or whole wheat waffle mix
2	tablespoons golden ground flaxseed
1	cup fat-free milk
4	egg whites
1/2	cup fat-free plain yogurt
1/2	cup water
1	tablespoon balsamic vinegar
10	teaspoons almond butter
2 1/2	pears, thinly sliced

1. Heat the waffle iron according to the manufacturer's directions.

2. Place the waffle mix in a large bowl. With a wooden spoon, make a "well" in the center of the mix. Add the flaxseed, milk, egg whites, yogurt, water, and vinegar to the well.

3. Stir in the wet ingredients, gradually incorporating the waffle mix, with about 10 turns of the spoon, or until a batter forms. Do not overmix.

4. Spoon 1/2 cup of the wet batter onto the waffle iron and close the lid. Cook for 3 to 4 minutes, or according to the waffle-iron directions. Transfer to cool on a wire rack.

5. Spread 2 teaspoons of the almond butter over half of 1 waffle. Top with 1/2 sliced pear and serve, or wrap in plastic wrap and store on the countertop for up to 2 hours. Repeat with the remaining waffles.

PER SERVING: 384 calories, 16 g protein, 63 g carbohydrates, 9 g fiber, 9 g fat (1 g saturated), 543 mg sodium

CHEF'S NOTE: These waffles freeze extremely well; just close without the filling in a zip-top bag and store in the freezer for up to 3 months.

ZUCCHINI-APPLE MUFFINS

Prep time: 15 minutes / Total time: 45 minutes /
Makes 12 muffins (2 muffins per serving)

1½ cups white whole wheat flour or whole wheat pastry flour

½ teaspoon baking soda

½ teaspoon baking powder

1 teaspoon pumpkin pie spice

1 teaspoon ground cinnamon

¼ teaspoon allspice

½ cup light brown sugar, packed

¼ cup unsalted butter

1½ cups grated zucchini (about 8 ounces)

1 apple, grated, including skin

1 cup 0% fat plain Greek yogurt

2 egg whites

¼ cup dried cherries

1. Heat the oven to 375°F. Line a 12-cup muffin tin with paper liners. Combine the flour, baking soda, baking powder, pumpkin pie spice, cinnamon, and allspice in a large bowl or zip-top bag. Stir or shake well to combine.

2. With a wooden spoon or an electric mixer on medium speed, mix the brown sugar and butter in a medium bowl until smooth.

3. Add the zucchini, apple, yogurt, egg whites, and cherries. Stir until just combined.

4. Add the flour mixture and stir about 10 strokes with a wooden spoon, or until a dense batter forms—don't overmix.

5. Fill the muffin papers to the top edge of the paper. Bake for 20 to 25 minutes, or until the center of a muffin springs back to the touch when pressed. Transfer to a wire rack to cool, then store in an airtight container for up to 3 days.

PER SERVING: 414 calories, 8 g protein, 76 g carbohydrates, 4 g fiber, 8 g fat (4 g saturated), 194 mg sodium

CHEF'S NOTE: Avoid stone ground whole wheat flour, which will make these muffins tough and grassy. White whole wheat and whole wheat pastry flour are more tender types of whole wheat flour. King Arthur and Arrowhead Mills, among other brands, make these types of flour.

You can substitute cranberries or raisins for the dried cherries, if you prefer. Have just one muffin for a 200-calorie snack.

Lunch

Soups, salads, and sandwiches are lunch staples for good reason—
they're all simple and portable ways to add Active Calories to your diet!
All of the following recipes provide around 400 calories and offer
chewy proteins and hearty fiber-rich foods. Men, remember that you
should add another 100 calories to each lunch.

CHICKEN MINESTRONE

Prep time: 10 minutes / Total time: 50 minutes / Serves 6 (2 cups per serving)

1	tablespoon olive oil
2	carrots, peeled and thinly sliced
2	celery stalks, thinly sliced
3	garlic cloves, minced
1	tablespoon rosemary, chopped
2	skinless chicken breasts on the bone
1	can or carton (32 ounces) low-sodium chicken broth
½	cup red wine
½	cup water
1	cup small whole wheat or brown rice pasta, such as shells
1	pound green beans or yellow wax beans, trimmed and cut into thirds
½	pound kale, thinly sliced
1	can (15 ounces) no-salt-added kidney or chickpeas, drained and well rinsed
¼	cup grated Parmesan cheese

1. Heat the oil in a large stockpot over medium-high heat. Add the carrots, celery, garlic, and rosemary. Cook for 3 to 4 minutes, stirring once or twice, or until the vegetables start to soften.

2. Add the chicken and broth, turning up the heat to high. Once the mixture comes to a boil, cover and turn the heat off. Let the chicken sit in the hot broth for 30 minutes, or until it's cooked through.

3. Remove the chicken to a plate to cool for 5 minutes, or until it is cool enough to shred.

4. Add the wine, water, and pasta to the stockpot and bring to a simmer. Cook for 10 minutes, or until the pasta is soft.

5. When the pasta is tender, add the green beans and kale and cook for 2 minutes longer, or until tender. Turn off the heat and return the chicken to the pot, along with the beans. Sprinkle with the cheese and serve immediately.

PER SERVING: 409 calories, 32 g protein, 49 g carbohydrates, 13 g fiber, 7 g fat (1 g saturated), 304 mg sodium

CHEF'S NOTE: You can substitute spinach or collard greens for the kale, if you prefer.

CARROT-GINGER SOUP
WITH CASHEWS AND CHICKEN

**Prep time: 10 minutes / Total time: 35 minutes /
Serves 4 (3 cups soup, including chicken and garnish, per serving)**

1	tablespoon olive oil
1	large white onion, peeled and chopped
3	garlic cloves, chopped
1	piece (3") fresh ginger, peeled and chopped
1½	pounds carrots (about 12 large carrots), peeled and chopped
4	cups low-sodium chicken broth
2	cups water
2	skinless chicken breasts on the bone
⅓	cup roasted, unsalted cashew pieces
¼	cup cilantro

1. Heat the oil in a large stockpot over medium heat. Add the onion, garlic, and ginger and cook for 3 to 4 minutes, or until the onion starts to soften.

2. Add the carrots, broth, water, and chicken breast. Bring to a simmer and cook for 15 minutes, or until the carrots are tender and the chicken is cooked through. Transfer the chicken to a plate.

3. Blend the soup using an immersion blender or food processor.

4. Shred the chicken and discard the bone.

5. Serve the soup topped with the shredded chicken, cashews, and cilantro.

PER SERVING: 401 calories, 26 g protein, 50 g carbohydrates, 7 g fiber, 11 g fat (2 g saturated), 514 mg sodium

CHEF'S NOTE: You can substitute basil or parsley for the cilantro, if you prefer.

MINI MEATBALL SOUP

Prep time: 15 minutes / Total time: 35 minutes /
Serves 4 (3 cups, including 10 meatballs, per serving)

2	garlic cloves
¼	cup grated Parmesan cheese
1	boneless, skinless chicken breast, cut into 4 pieces
1	cup whole wheat bread crumbs
2	tablespoons fat-free milk
1	egg
¼	teaspoon ground black pepper
4	teaspoons olive oil
2	small carrots, peeled and chopped, about 1 cup
2	celery stalks, chopped
1	small onion, peeled and chopped
1	piece (1") fresh ginger, peeled and chopped
1	can (15 ounces) no-salt-added chopped tomatoes
1	can (15 ounces) reduced-sodium chicken broth
1	cup water
1	cup small whole wheat pasta
1	cup frozen peas or edamame
1	cup frozen green beans

1. Place the garlic and cheese in a food processor and pulse until the garlic is chopped. Add the chicken, bread crumbs, milk, egg, and pepper.

2. Form the mixture into small meatballs about the size of a grape and place on a sheet of wax paper (you should have about 40 total).

3. Heat a large stockpot over high heat and add 2 teaspoons of the oil. Add the meatballs and brown for 3 to 4 minutes, turning occasionally. Transfer the meatballs to a plate.

4. Add the remaining 2 teaspoons oil and the carrots, celery, onion, and ginger. Cook over medium heat for 3 to 4 minutes, or until the vegetables start to soften.

5. Add the tomatoes, broth, water, and pasta. Cover and reduce to a simmer. Cook for 8 to 10 minutes, or until the pasta is soft.

6. Return the meatballs to the soup and add the peas or edamame and green beans. Simmer for another 2 minutes, or until the peas are warm, and serve immediately.

PER SERVING: 412 calories, 24 g protein, 56 g carbohydrates, 10 g fiber, 10 g fat (2 g saturated), 576 mg sodium

EGG SALAD

Prep time: 5 minutes / **Total time:** 45 minutes / **Serves** 4 (1 wrap with 1 cup of filling)

8	eggs
1	package (8 ounces) frozen artichokes, thawed
¼	cup 0% fat plain Greek yogurt
¼	cup chopped parsley
3	tablespoons light mayonnaise
2	tablespoons dried onion
2	tablespoons sweet pickle relish
4	8" whole grain wraps
8	lettuce leaves, such as butter or romaine

1. Place the eggs in a medium saucepan and cover with cold water. Bring to a boil over high heat, then immediately turn off the heat. Rest for 15 minutes, covered. Drain the eggs and run under cold water. Peel the eggs and discard all the yolks except for 2.

2. Chop the whites of the eggs and add them to a large bowl, along with the yolks. Add the artichokes, yogurt, parsley, mayonnaise, dried onion, and relish. Stir until well combined.

3. Divide the mixture among the wraps and top with the lettuce leaves. Fold over the sides and roll to close. Serve immediately or wrap in aluminum foil and refrigerate until ready to serve.

PER SERVING: 375 calories, 19 g protein, 48 g carbohydrates, 12 g fiber, 10 g fat (2 g saturated), 652 mg sodium

CALIFORNIA SALAD

Prep time: 15 minutes / Total time: 30 minutes /
Serves 4 (3 cups salad, including all the toppings, per serving)

2	raw chicken cutlets (about ½ pound)
1	teaspoon mild chili powder
1	teaspoon garlic powder
¼	teaspoon freshly ground black pepper
1	tablespoon olive oil
4	slices nitrate-free turkey bacon, chopped
2	tablespoons honey
2	tablespoons apple cider or malt vinegar
2	teaspoons Dijon mustard
8	cups chopped fresh romaine lettuce (about 3 medium heads)
1	pound tomatoes, chopped
4	scallions, thinly sliced
⅓	cup shredded low-fat Cheddar cheese
	Whole grain or multigrain English muffins, toasted

1. Sprinkle the cutlets with the chili powder, garlic powder, and pepper.

2. Heat the oil in a large skillet over high heat. Immediately add the chicken and cook for 8 to 10 minutes, or until no longer pink in the center, turning once throughout cooking. Transfer to a shallow bowl.

3. Add the bacon to the skillet and cook for 2 to 4 minutes over medium heat, or until crisp. Turn off the heat and add the honey, vinegar, mustard, and any juices from the resting chicken.

4. Whisk the dressing directly in the skillet and add 1 tablespoon water if the dressing ingredients don't combine easily.

5. Slice the chicken into strips.

6. Place the lettuce in a large bowl, along with the tomatoes, scallions, and cheese. Drizzle with the dressing from the skillet and toss well. Serve immediately with the English muffins.

PER SERVING: 415 calories, 26 g protein, 52 g carbohydrates, 8 g fiber, 14 g fat (3 g saturated), 713 mg sodium

CHEF'S NOTE: You can substitute shallots for the scallions, if you prefer.

TACO SALAD

**Prep time: 10 minutes / Total time: 25 minutes /
Serves 4 (1 whole wheat tortilla "bowl" with 2½ cups filling per serving)**

1	cup jarred salsa verde
1	medium zucchini (stem removed), cut into quarters
1	tablespoon olive oil
2	boneless, skinless chicken breasts, cubed
4	low-fat whole wheat tortillas (10" diameter)
6	cups shredded romaine lettuce
1½	cups no-salt-added canned kidney or black beans, rinsed and drained
4	tablespoons low-fat sour cream
4	tablespoons grated low-fat Cheddar or pepper Jack cheese
4	teaspoons hot sauce

1. Preheat the oven to 400°F. Place the salsa verde in a blender or food processor, along with the zucchini. Process or blend until a chunky sauce forms. Add a few tablespoons of water if the mixture doesn't blend properly. Set aside.

2. Heat a large oven-safe skillet over high heat and add the oil. Add the chicken and cook for 2 to 3 minutes, turning once or twice, or until the chicken begins to brown.

3. Add the salsa verde mixture to the skillet and decrease the heat to low. Slide the skillet into the oven.

4. Coat 4 oven-safe 2-cup bowls with cooking spray. Press 1 tortilla into each bowl and bake, along with the chicken, for 8 to 10 minutes, or until the tortillas are crisp. Remove from the bowls and set aside.

5. Check the chicken pieces to be sure they are cooked through, baking for 5 minutes longer if necessary.

6. Divide the lettuce, beans, chicken mixture, sour cream, cheese, and hot sauce among the tortilla shells and serve immediately.

PER SERVING: 401 calories, 27 g protein, 47 g carbohydrates, 9 g fiber, 10 g fat (3 g saturated), 720 mg sodium

CHEF'S NOTE: If you want to take this lunch to go, cook the chicken and the tortilla shells separately. Reheat the chicken mixture and fill the tortilla shells just before eating.

TUNA SALAD CRUNCH

Prep time: 5 minutes / Total time: 10 minutes /
Serves 4 (1 cup tuna salad plus 2 slices bread per serving)

¼ cup light mayonnaise

2 tablespoons 0% fat plain Greek yogurt

¼ teaspoon freshly ground black pepper

2 cans (5 ounces each) tuna in spring water, drained

1 can (15 ounces) no-salt-added cannellini beans, rinsed and drained

½ cup mint, chopped

4 jalapeño chile peppers, seeded and chopped

½ cup wasabi peas or dried soybeans

4 small whole wheat pitas (6″ diameter), cut in half

1. Place the mayonnaise, yogurt, and black pepper in a large bowl. Whisk until smooth.

2. Fold in the tuna, beans, mint, chile peppers, and wasabi peas or soybeans.

3. Distribute the filling evenly among the pitas and serve.

PER SERVING: 381 calories, 28 g protein, 47 g carbohydrates, 10 g fiber, 10 g fat (2 g saturated), 561 mg sodium

CHEF'S NOTE: If you aren't serving this immediately, pack the wasabi peas separately and stir into the mix just before serving. Otherwise they will soften and you won't get that satisfying (and chewy) crunch.

BARBECUE CHICKEN SALAD

**Prep time: 5 minutes / Total time: 10 minutes /
Serves 4 (2½ cups lentils with chicken per serving)**

1	cup French or green lentils, rinsed
2½	cups water
1	chipotle chile in adobo sauce
1	tablespoon adobo sauce
¼	cup walnuts, toasted and chopped
4	stalks celery, chopped
1	bunch asparagus (about 1½ pounds), cut into 1" pieces
2	grilled chicken breasts, sliced
½	cup jarred barbecue sauce

1. Place the lentils, water, chipotle chile, and adobo sauce in a rice cooker and set to cook. Or, if you don't have a rice cooker, place the lentils, water, chipotle chile, and adobo sauce in a small saucepan, bring to a boil, and cover. Reduce to a simmer for 10 to 15 minutes, or until most of the water is gone and the lentils are almost cooked through.

2. If using the rice cooker, add the asparagus as soon as the cooker shuts off and steam for 5 minutes. If using the saucepan, add the asparagus once most of the water is gone and cook for 5 minutes longer, or until the asparagus is tender. Remove the lentil mixture from the rice cooker or saucepan and place in a bowl, uncovered.

3. Place the chicken in a medium bowl and add the walnuts, celery, and barbecue sauce. Stir to coat. Transfer the lentil mixture to a platter and top with the chicken.

PER SERVING: 401 calories, 34 g protein, 48 g carbohydrates, 11 g fiber, 9 g fat (0 g saturated), 528 mg sodium

CHEF'S NOTE: If you can't find chipotle chile in adobo sauce in your supermarket, you can mail-order a jar; it's not expensive. Freeze the chiles you don't use in a zip-top bag. Or mash together garlic and red-pepper flakes with 1 tablespoon tomato paste and use that instead. It won't have quite the same heat and texture as the chipotle chile but will give you a reasonable approximation.

AVOCADO SEAFOOD SALAD

Prep time: 10 minutes / Total time: 20 minutes / Serves 4 (2 cups per serving)

1	teaspoon canola or light olive oil
1	pound shrimp, peeled and deveined
$\frac{1}{4}$	teaspoon cayenne
$\frac{1}{8}$	teaspoon freshly ground black pepper
2	large pink grapefruit
5	ounces baby spinach
$1\frac{1}{2}$	Hass avocados, chopped
2	stalks celery, chopped
1	small shallot, minced
1	teaspoon Dijon mustard
2	teaspoons honey
2	pitas ($6\frac{1}{2}$" diameter), cut in half

1. Heat a large skillet over high heat and add the oil. Sprinkle the shrimp with the cayenne and pepper and add to the skillet. Reduce the heat to medium. Cook for 4 to 6 minutes, stirring occasionally, or until pink and no longer translucent inside.

2. Cut the bottom and top of the peel off each grapefruit to make a flat surface. Set one of the flat sides on a cutting board and trim away the remaining peel. Holding each grapefruit over a medium bowl to catch the juice, separate the grapefruit sections from the white membrane with a small paring knife, letting them fall into the bowl. Scoop out the sections and transfer to a large bowl, along with the spinach, avocados, and celery. Set aside.

3. Add the shallot, mustard, and honey to the medium bowl with the grapefruit juice. Whisk until smooth. Drizzle the dressing over the bowl containing the spinach and add the shrimp. Toss and serve each portion of salad with a pita half.

PER SERVING: 398 calories, 29 g protein, 47 g carbohydrates, 9 g fiber, 12 g fat (2 g saturated), 447 mg sodium

TROPICAL SALAD

Prep time: 5 minutes / Total time: 15 minutes /
Serves 4 (2 cups salad plus 16 crackers per serving)

½	teaspoon canola oil
3	tablespoons chopped pecans
1	teaspoon curry powder
1	teaspoon packed light brown sugar
1	teaspoon hot sauce
4	boneless, skinless chicken breasts, grilled, cut into strips
2	mangoes, peeled and cubed
2	bananas, sliced
1	large head romaine lettuce, sliced
¼	red onion, minced
	Juice of 1 lime
1	teaspoon curry powder
¼	teaspoon salt
52	whole wheat crackers

1. Heat the oil in a small skillet over medium heat. Add the pecans, curry powder, brown sugar, and hot sauce. Cook for 2 to 3 minutes, stirring often, or until the brown sugar coats the nuts and the spices become fragrant. Turn off the heat and set aside.

2. Place the chicken, mangoes, bananas, and lettuce in a large bowl.

3. Place the onion, lime juice, curry powder, and salt in a small bowl and whisk. Drizzle the dressing over the chicken mixture and top with the pecans. Toss well to combine and serve immediately with the crackers.

PER SERVING: 398 calories, 19 g protein, 57 g carbohydrates, 7 g fiber, 12 g fat (1 g saturated), 439 mg sodium

{ CHEF'S NOTE: If you're not planning to eat the salad right away, don't add the bananas. Store the salad and dressing in separate containers; then, right before eating, add the bananas to the salad and drizzle with the dressing.

SIX-INCH LUNCH SUB

Prep time: 5 minutes / Total time: 10 minutes / Serves 1

2	tablespoons balsamic vinegar
1	teaspoon olive oil
1/4	teaspoon freshly ground black pepper
1	piece (6") whole wheat baguette (about 2 ounces)
1	slice low-fat Swiss cheese
1/2	grilled chicken breast
1	cup baby spinach
1/2	cup thinly sliced red bell pepper

1. Place the vinegar, oil, and black pepper in a small bowl and whisk well to combine.

2. Drizzle over the inside of the baguette. Add the cheese, chicken, spinach, and bell pepper.

3. Wrap the sandwich in plastic wrap or aluminum foil. Serve immediately or refrigerate for up to 1 day before serving.

PER SERVING: 381 calories, 25 g protein, 52 g carbohydrates, 6 g fiber, 12 g fat (2 g saturated), 670 mg sodium

CHEF'S NOTE: Pickled peppers would be a delicious addition and would add warming Active Calories through the vinegar in the pickling solution, but they tend to be high in sodium. This recipe is already relatively high in sodium because of the bread and cheese, so if you really want to add pickles of some sort, consider leaving off the cheese.

SPICY CHICKEN TACOS

**Prep time: 10 minutes / Total time: 40 minutes /
Serves 4 (3 tacos with 1 cup filling per serving)**

2	teaspoons olive oil
1	pound boneless, skinless chicken breasts (about 3), trimmed and cut into strips
1	carrot, grated
1	stalk celery, thinly sliced
2	garlic cloves, chopped
2	teaspoons cornstarch
1	teaspoon ground cumin
1	teaspoon ground mild chili powder
1/4	teaspoon cayenne
2	tablespoons pickled jalapeño chile peppers, chopped
1/2	cup water
12	soft whole grain flour tortillas (8" diameter)
1/2	cup shredded 2% reduced-fat Cheddar cheese
4	large romaine lettuce leaves, thinly sliced
1/4	cup reduced-fat sour cream
1/2	cup jarred medium salsa

1. Coat a large skillet with cooking spray and heat over medium-high heat. Add the oil.

2. Add the chicken, carrot, celery, and garlic. Cook for 10 to 15 minutes, stirring occasionally, or until the chicken begins to brown and the vegetables soften.

3. Sprinkle with the cornstarch, cumin, chili powder, and cayenne. Continue to cook for 1 minute longer, or until the spices become fragrant.

4. Add the chile peppers and water. Reduce to a simmer and cook for 5 to 10 minutes, or until the chicken is no longer pink in the center and a thick sauce forms.

5. Meanwhile, place the tortillas in the oven or toaster oven, heated to 350°F, for 10 minutes, or until warm. Assemble the tacos by spooning 1/3 cup of the filling into each tortilla. Divide the lettuce, cheese, sour cream, and salsa evenly among the tortillas. Fold over and serve immediately.

PER SERVING: 400 calories, 36 g protein, 32g carbohydrates, 17 g fiber, 12 g fat (3 g saturated), 772 mg sodium

STEAK BURRITO

Prep time: 5 minutes / Total time: 20 minutes /
Serves 4 (1 whole wheat tortilla plus 1½ cups filling per serving)

½ pound flank steak, sliced

1 chipotle chile in adobo sauce, chopped

1 tablespoon adobo sauce

2 garlic cloves, minced

1 teaspoon fresh thyme

2 cups broccoli florets, chopped

2 cups baby spinach, chopped

4 large whole wheat tortillas (8" diameter)

2 tomatoes, chopped

4 tablespoons jarred spicy tomato salsa

1. Place the steak in an 8" × 12" dish. Rub with the chile, adobo sauce, garlic, and thyme. Cover and refrigerate for at least 2 hours.

2. Preheat the oven to 350°F. Wrap the tortillas in aluminum foil and warm in the oven for 10 minutes.

3. Meanwhile, heat a grill or large skillet over high heat. Coat with cooking spray and then add the steak. Cook for 4 to 5 minutes, or until the meat is still slightly pink but not translucent. Transfer to a bowl.

4. Place the broccoli on the griddle and cook for 1 to 2 minutes, or until it softens. Add the spinach and turn until it wilts. Transfer the broccoli and spinach to the bowl with the meat and toss to mix.

5. Set out the tortillas and top each with one-quarter of the mixture. Top each with 1 tablespoon of the tomatoes and salsa. Fold in the sides of each tortilla and roll to form a burrito. Serve immediately or wrap in aluminum foil and refrigerate until ready to serve.

PER SERVING: 383 calories, 25 g protein, 37 g carbohydrates, 12 g fiber, 12 g fat (2 g saturated), 558 mg sodium

CHEF'S NOTE: If you double this recipe, you can use the leftovers for the Steak Sandwich with Peppers and Onions on page 140.

CUBAN SANDWICH

Prep time: 5 minutes / Total time: 20 minutes / Serves 1

1	large portobello mushroom, stem removed
½	teaspoon olive oil
1	small red onion, peeled and sliced
1	tablespoon 0% fat plain Greek yogurt
1	tablespoon light mayonnaise
1	tablespoon sweet pickle relish
1	piece (6") whole wheat baguette, cut in half (about 2 ounces)
2	ounces lean pork loin, sliced
1	slice low-sodium baked ham

1. With a teaspoon, scrape the underside of the mushroom to remove the black gills. Discard the gills.

2. Heat a griddle or large skillet over high heat. Add the oil, mushroom, and onion. Cook for 8 to 10 minutes, stirring and turning occasionally, or until the onion begins to brown and the mushroom is cooked through. Add 1 tablespoon water if the onion begins to stick.

3. Spread the yogurt, mayo, and relish on 1 side of the baguette and top with the pork and ham. Spoon the onion on top. Cut the mushroom in half and layer it on top of the onion.

4. Top with the remaining piece of baguette and return the sandwich to the griddle or skillet.

5. Place a sandwich press or another heavy pot on top to compress the sandwich. Remove the sandwich press or heavy pot and cook over low heat for 1 minute total, turning the sandwich once, or until it browns lightly. Serve immediately or wrap in aluminum foil and refrigerate until ready to serve.

PER SERVING: 394 calories, 24 g protein, 52 g carbohydrates, 6 g fiber, 9 g fat (1g saturated), 749 mg sodium

PULLED BBQ CHICKEN SANDWICH

Prep time: 5 minutes / Total time: 45 minutes / Serves 4 (1 sandwich per serving)

2   boneless, skinless chicken breasts

1   tablespoon olive oil

1   large onion, peeled and thinly sliced

2   large tomatoes (about 12 ounces), chopped

¼   cup water

½   cup jarred barbecue sauce

4   small whole wheat hoagie rolls

2   large carrots, peeled and shredded

2   cups shredded red cabbage

2   tablespoons light mayo

2   tablespoons 0% fat plain Greek yogurt

1. Fill a medium pot with water and bring to a boil. Add the chicken and cover with a lid. Turn off the heat and let the chicken rest in the hot water for at least 30 minutes, or until it is cooked all the way through. Transfer the chicken to a cutting board and discard the water.

2. Heat the oil in a large skillet over medium heat. Add the onion and cook for 6 to 7 minutes, or until the onion begins to brown and is soft.

3. Add the tomatoes and water and cook for 3 to 4 minutes longer, or until the tomatoes give off their liquid.

4. Stir in the barbecue sauce and turn off the heat. Shred the chicken with your fingers and add it to the skillet. Stir until the sauce coats the chicken. Divide the chicken among the rolls.

5. Place the carrots, cabbage, mayo, and yogurt in a large bowl. Toss to coat, divide among the 4 sandwiches, and serve immediately or wrap. Refrigerate for up to 1 day until ready to enjoy.

PER SERVING: 404 calories, 22 g protein, 59 g carbohydrates, 8 g fiber, 9 g fat (1 g saturated), 649 mg sodium

BLACK BEAN BURGER

Prep time: 5 minutes / Total time: 20 minutes / Serves 4 (1 burger per serving)

1	can (15 ounces) no-salt-added black beans, rinsed and drained
6	ounces mushrooms, quartered
½	red onion, quartered
6	tablespoons whole wheat bread crumbs
¼	cup cilantro, chopped
2	garlic cloves, minced
2	teaspoons low-sodium soy sauce
1	jalapeño chile pepper, seeded
1	egg white
1	tablespoon canola oil
4	slices low-fat cheese, such as pepper Jack or mozzarella
4	small whole wheat sandwich rolls, toasted
4	lettuce leaves
1	small tomato, cut into 4 thick slices

1. Place the beans, mushrooms, onion, bread crumbs, cilantro, garlic, soy sauce, chile pepper, and egg white in a food processor. Blend until a smooth mixture forms. Separate into 4 equal mounds and form each into a burger.

2. Heat a large skillet over medium heat and add the oil. Cook the burgers for 4 to 5 minutes, turning once.

3. Top each burger with a slice of cheese and slide into the oven. Bake for 5 to 6 minutes, or until the burger is warm.

4. Transfer to the burgers to the buns and top with lettuce and tomato. Serve immediately.

PER SERVING: 406 calories, 21 g protein, 51 g carbohydrates, 11 g fiber, 13 g fat (5 g saturated), 680 mg sodium

CHEF'S NOTE: Any hot pepper can be substituted for the chile pepper, if you prefer.

STEAK SANDWICH WITH PEPPERS AND ONIONS

Prep time: 5 minutes / Total time: 10 minutes /
Serves 4 (1 sandwich with 1½ cups filling per serving)

½	pound flank steak, thinly sliced
2	garlic cloves, minced
2	tablespoons cilantro leaves, chopped
1	red onion, peeled and thinly sliced
1	green bell pepper, seeded and thinly sliced
1	poblano or Cubanelle pepper, thinly sliced
¼	teaspoon salt
4	slices reduced-fat provolone or Swiss cheese
4	whole wheat sandwich rolls
1	head romaine lettuce, chopped

1. Place the steak, garlic, and cilantro in a medium bowl and toss to coat.

2. Heat a large griddle or skillet over high heat. Coat with cooking spray and add the steak. Cook for 3 to 4 minutes, turning twice, or until the steak is lightly brown on the edges but still pink in the center. Transfer to a plate.

3. Coat the skillet with another layer of cooking spray and add the onion, bell pepper, and poblano or Cubanelle pepper. Sprinkle with the salt. Reduce the heat to medium and cook for 6 to 7 minutes, turning often, or until the peppers are soft.

4. Place 1 cheese slice into each roll and heat in a toasted oven or an oven preheated to 350°F for 5 minutes.

5. Add the steak, onion-and-pepper mixture, and lettuce and serve immediately.

PER SERVING: 367 calories, 25 g protein, 40 g carbohydrates, 6 g fiber, 13 g fat (6 g saturated), 735 mg sodium

CHEF'S NOTE: You can substitute 2 large jalapeño chile peppers for the poblano or Cubanelle pepper, if you prefer.

You can use steak left over from the Steak Burrito recipe on page 136 for this, if you have any.

PEPPERONI CALZONE

Prep time: 10 minutes / Total time: 40 minutes / Serves 4 (1 calzone per serving)

1	can (15 ounces) no-salt-added chopped tomatoes
1	teaspoon olive oil
1	sprig basil
1	pound store-bought raw whole wheat pizza dough, thawed
16	slices turkey pepperoni (about 1^1/$_2$ ounces)
^{1}/$_2$	cup shredded reduced-fat mozzarella cheese
^{1}/$_2$	cup part-skim ricotta cheese
2	cups broccoli florets, chopped
5	ounces mushrooms, sliced

1. Preheat the oven to 400°F. Place the tomatoes, oil, and basil in a blender and blend until smooth.

2. Cut the pizza dough into 4 equal pieces and roll them out into 8" circles. Transfer to 2 baking sheets, 2 dough disks per sheet.

3. Place 4 pieces of the pepperoni in the center of each dough disk. Spoon a quarter of the sauce on top of the pepperoni and then distribute the mozzarella, ricotta, broccoli, and mushrooms. Fold the dough over to make a pocket and press closed with the tines of a fork.

4. Bake for 15 to 20 minutes, or until the dough is cooked through and the tops of the calzones are lightly browned. Serve immediately.

PER SERVING: 391 calories, 21 g protein, 56 g carbohydrates, 10 g fiber, 11 g fat (2 g saturated), 883 mg sodium

SHRIMP COCKTAIL ON TOAST

Prep time: 5 minutes / Total time: 15 minutes /
Serves 4 (6 toast slices with topping per serving)

1   small whole wheat baguette (10 ounces), cut into ½" slices

2   garlic cloves, cut in half

1   tablespoon olive oil

½   pound medium shrimp, peeled, deveined, and chopped

1   ripe Hass avocado

2   tomatoes, chopped

1   package (9 ounces) frozen artichokes, thawed

2   tablespoons cocktail sauce

Juice of 1 lemon

1. Heat a grill or large skillet over medium heat. Rub the bread slices with the garlic and coat with cooking spray. Place on a grill or in a skillet and toast for 3 to 4 minutes per side, or until golden. Set aside.

2. Chop the garlic cloves. Heat a large skillet over high heat. Add the oil, shrimp, and garlic. Cook for 4 to 5 minutes, stirring often, or until the shrimp turn pink and are cooked through.

3. Transfer to a large bowl, along with the avocado, tomatoes, artichokes, cocktail sauce, and lemon juice. Toss until the sauce coats the shrimp and vegetables. Top each slice of toast with 2 heaping tablespoons of the shrimp mixture and serve immediately.

PER SERVING: 390 calories, 56 g protein, 56 g carbohydrates, 12 g fiber, 10 g fat (1 g saturated), 659 mg sodium

PIZZETTE WITH ARRABIATA SAUCE

**Prep time: 10 minutes / Total time: 40 minutes /
Serves 4 (1 pizzette with small salad per serving)**

1	tablespoon olive oil
1	jalapeño chile pepper or Holland pepper, chopped
1	garlic clove, minced
1	can (15 ounces) diced tomatoes
¼	cup wine
4	whole wheat pitas (6″ diameter)
½	cup grated part-skim mozzarella cheese
8	ounces mixed greens
2	tomatoes, chopped
2	carrots, peeled and chopped
½	cup bottled light salad dressing

1. Warm the oil a small saucepan over medium heat. Add the pepper and garlic and cook for 2 to 3 minutes, stirring occasionally, or until the garlic begins to turn golden.

2. Reduce the heat to low and add the diced tomatoes and wine. Cook for 10 to 15 minutes longer, stirring occasionally, or until the tomatoes begin to break apart. Set aside.

3. Preheat the oven to 400°F. Line a baking sheet with aluminum foil. Place the pitas on the baking sheet and top each with a quarter of the sauce. Sprinkle with the cheese and bake for 7 to 8 minutes, or until the cheese is bubbly and begins to brown.

4. Place the greens, chopped tomatoes, carrots, and dressing in a large bowl. Toss to coat. Serve alongside the pizzettes.

PER SERVING: 381 calories, 15 g protein, 53 g carbohydrates, 10 g fiber, 12 g fat (1 g saturated), 514 mg sodium

TWICE-COOKED POTATO SKINS

Prep time: 15 minutes / Total time: 45 minutes /
Serves 4 (4 potato skins with filling, along with 2 cups romaine lettuce per serving)

4	large baking potatoes, such as Idaho (about 2 pounds)
2	cups baby spinach, thinly sliced
1/2	cup 0% fat plain Greek yogurt
1/3	cup reduced-fat sour cream
1	teaspoon hot sauce
1	tablespoon olive oil
4	ounces nitrate-free turkey bacon, chopped
1/4	pound 7% lean ground turkey
1/2	teaspoon garlic powder
2	tablespoons dried onion
1/2	cup crumbled feta cheese
4	scallions, thinly sliced
8	cups shredded romaine lettuce

1. Fill a large stockpot with 3" water. Bring to a boil. Add the potatoes and cook for 15 minutes, or until fork-tender.

2. Remove the potatoes and transfer to a cutting board. Cut in half lengthwise, scoop out the centers, and place the filling into a large bowl.

3. Add the spinach, yogurt, sour cream, and hot sauce. Mash with a fork to break up the potatoes until fairly smooth and set aside.

4. Preheat the oven to 400°F. Warm the oil in a medium skillet over medium heat. Add the skins and cook for 2 to 3 minutes per side, or until brown. Transfer to a baking sheet lined with aluminum foil.

5. In the same skillet, add the bacon, turkey, garlic powder, and dried onion. Cook for 4 to 5 minutes, stirring often with a wooden spoon and breaking up the turkey, or until it is brown and no longer pink.

6. Spoon the turkey mixture over the hollow side of the skins. Top with the mashed-potato mixture and scatter with the cheese and scallions. Bake for 10 to 15 minutes, or until the topping is hot. Serve immediately over the lettuce.

PER SERVING: 398 calories, 32 g protein, 25 g carbohydrates, 5 g fiber, 11 g fat (4 g saturated), 539 mg sodium

CHEF'S NOTE: Dried onions can be found in the spice aisle; they're inexpensive and add a lot of texture and flavor with no added salt or sugar.
    This is a great dish for anyone who craves "meat and potatoes."

CHILI-TOPPED SWEET POTATO

Prep time: 5 minutes / Total time: 35 minutes /
Serves 4 (1½ cups chili with ½ sweet potato per serving)

2	teaspoons olive oil
½	pound ground sirloin
2	garlic cloves, minced
¼	teaspoon salt
1	teaspoon cumin
1	teaspoon mild chili powder
2	cups low-sodium beef broth
½	cup water
1	tablespoon ground flaxseed
1	lime, zested and juiced
1	chipotle chile in adobo sauce
1	teaspoon adobo sauce
1	cup whole wheat or brown rice pasta
2	large sweet potatoes (about 12 ounces)
4	tablespoons reduced-fat sour cream

1. Heat a large stockpot over medium-high heat. Add the oil. Add the sirloin, garlic, and salt and cook for 1 minute without stirring. Cook for 4 to 5 minutes longer, stirring occasionally, or until the meat is browned.

2. Sprinkle the meat with the cumin and chili powder. Cook for 1 minute longer, or until the spices are fragrant.

3. Add the broth, water, flaxseed, lime zest and juice, chipotle chile, and adobo sauce to the stockpot. Bring to a boil and then immediately reduce to a simmer.

4. Add the pasta and cook covered for 20 to 25 minutes, or until the pasta is cooked through.

5. Score the sweet potatoes with the tines of a fork. Wrap each potato in a paper towel. Microwave on high for 4 to 5 minutes, or until the potato is soft to the touch.

6. Cut 1 potato in half lengthwise and place in a soup bowl. Top with 1½ cups of the chili and a dollop of the sour cream. Repeat with the remaining potato and serve immediately.

PER SERVING: 387 calories, 24 g protein, 48 g carbohydrates, 6 g fiber, 12 g fat (4 g saturated), 402 mg sodium

CHEF'S NOTE: You can cook the sweet potato ahead of time.

PAPRIKA CHICKEN AND BISCUITS

Prep time: 10 minutes / Total time: 40 minutes /
Serves 6 (2 cups stew plus 1 large biscuit per serving)

1	tablespoon olive oil
1	small onion, chopped
2	garlic cloves, minced
1	tablespoon whole wheat flour
1	tablespoon paprika
1½	cups fat-free milk
1	cup low-sodium chicken broth
4	carrots, peeled and chopped
1	cup frozen peas
4	boneless, skinless chicken breasts, cut into 1" cubes
2	tablespoons half-and-half
1	box (8.5 ounces) cornbread mix
1	egg

1. Preheat the oven to 400°F. Heat the oil in a large stockpot over medium heat. Add the onion and garlic and cook for 4 to 5 minutes, stirring occasionally, or until the onion softens.

2. Add the flour and paprika and reduce the heat to low. Cook for 1 minute longer, stirring often, as the flour coats the onion mixture and the inside of the pan.

3. Whisk in 1 cup of the milk and the broth. Bring to a boil and then immediately reduce to a simmer.

4. Add the carrots and cook for 3 to 4 minutes, uncovered, or until the carrots are almost tender.

5. Stir in the peas, chicken, and half-and-half. Simmer for 1 minute longer while you make the biscuit topping.

6. Place the cornbread mix in a medium bowl, along with the egg and remaining ½ cup milk. Stir with a wooden spoon until just incorporated.

7. Spoon the corn batter over the top of the chicken stew and transfer to the oven. Bake for 15 to 20 minutes, uncovered, or until the biscuits have puffed and the chicken is cooked through.

PER SERVING: 382 calories, 28 g protein, 43 g carbohydrates, 5 g fiber, 10 g fat (2 g saturated), 631 mg sodium

CHEF'S NOTE: You can substitute lima beans for the peas, if you prefer.

STRAWBERRY SALMON

Prep time: 5 minutes / Total time: 30 minutes /
Serves 4 (4-ounce piece of salmon and 1½ cups couscous with green beans per serving)

1	pound boneless salmon fillets, skin on
½	teaspoon salt
¼	teaspoon freshly cracked black pepper
⅛	teaspoon cayenne
1	teaspoon olive oil
1	large shallot or ½ small red onion, minced
1	pound green beans, chopped
¾	cup whole wheat couscous
1½	cups + 2 tablespoons water
1	lemon, juiced
1	pint strawberries
2	tablespoons balsamic vinegar
1	teaspoon sugar

1. Preheat the oven to 400°F. Place the salmon, skin side down, in an 8″ × 12″ baking dish. Sprinkle the tops of the fillets with the salt, pepper, and cayenne. Coat with a thin layer of cooking spray and transfer to the oven. Bake for 12 to 15 minutes, or until the salmon is cooked through and no longer translucent in the center.

2. Heat the oil in a small stockpot over medium heat. Add the shallot or onion and cook for 2 to 3 minutes, or until it begins to brown.

3. Add the green beans and cook for 1 minute longer, covered, or until they turn a shade darker.

4. Add the couscous and 1½ cups of the water. Bring to a boil and stir in half the lemon juice. Turn off the heat and cover for 15 minutes. Fluff before serving.

5. Place the strawberries, vinegar, remaining 2 tablespoons water, sugar, and remaining lemon juice in a small saucepan. Bring to a simmer and cook for 10 minutes, or until the strawberries are soft and a syrupy sauce forms. Serve immediately on top of the salmon, along with the couscous.

PER SERVING: 399 calories, 29 g protein, 66 g carbohydrates, 8 g fiber, 14 g fat (2 g saturated), 371 mg sodium

SPANISH CHICKEN AND RICE

Prep time: 10 minutes / Total time: 1 hour / Serves 4 (2½ cups per serving)

1	tablespoon olive oil
1	onion, chopped
⅓	cup oil-cured olives
½	cup chopped cilantro
½	cup chopped parsley
2	garlic cloves, chopped
1	tablespoon chopped chipotle chile in adobo sauce
1	cup uncooked short-grain brown rice
1	can (28 ounces) no-salt-added tomatoes
1	can (15 ounces) low-sodium chicken broth
3	boneless, skinless chicken breasts

1. Heat the oil in a large stockpot over medium heat. Add the onion, olives, cilantro, parsley, and garlic. Cook for 4 to 5 minutes, stirring often, or until the mixture is fragrant and the herbs have wilted.

2. Add the chipotle chile and cook for 1 minute longer.

3. Add the rice and stir to coat in oil. Add the tomatoes and broth and bring to a boil. Reduce to a simmer, cover, and cook for 15 minutes.

4. Add the chicken. Cover and cook for 20 to 25 minutes longer, or until the rice is cooked through and the chicken is no longer pink when cut with a knife. Remove the chicken from the pot and place on a cutting board. Cook the stew for 5 to 10 minutes longer, or until the rice is cooked through. Shred the chicken and return to the stew. Serve immediately or cool before transferring to an airtight container.

PER SERVING: 397 calories, 28 g protein, 46 g carbohydrates, 3 g fiber, 9 g fat (1 g saturated), 571 mg sodium

CHEF'S NOTE: You can substitute parsley for the cilantro, if you prefer.

MISO BEEF AND NOODLES

Prep time: 5 minutes / Total time: 25 minutes /
Serves 4 (3 cups, including noodles and beef, per serving)

½ pound flank steak, thinly sliced

2 tablespoons mellow white miso paste

4 garlic cloves, minced

¼ cup cilantro, chopped

1 tablespoon canola oil

2 carrots, peeled and thinly sliced

4 scallions, chopped

½ pound shiitake mushrooms, thinly sliced (discard stems)

2 cups low-sodium beef broth

2 cups water

6 ounces Asian noodles, such as udon or ramen, cooked according to package directions

2 cups packed baby spinach leaves

1. Place the flank steak on a plate. Rub the miso, garlic, and cilantro over the meat and set aside.

2. Heat a large stockpot over high heat. Add the oil. Add the steak and cook for 2 to 3 minutes, or until the meat begins to brown on the outside but is still pink. Transfer to a plate.

3. Add the carrots, scallions, and mushrooms and continue to cook over high heat for 3 to 4 minutes, stirring often, or until the mushrooms start to soften. Add the broth and water.

4. Reduce the heat to low, add the noodles, and cover. Cook for 2 to 3 minutes longer, stirring occasionally, or until the noodles are cooked through.

5. Add the spinach leaves, which will wilt immediately. Return the meat to the pot and serve immediately.

PER SERVING: 398 calories, 25 g protein, 56 g carbohydrates, 7 g fiber, 8 g fat (1 g saturated), 659 mg sodium

CHEF'S NOTE: You can substitute any kind of mushroom for the shiitake, if you prefer.

SESAME-TUNA BENTO BOX

Prep time: 5 minutes / Total time: 40 minutes /
Serves 4 (2 ounces tuna, 1 cup mushroom rice, and 1 cup broccoli per serving)

2	teaspoons butter
1/2	pound shiitake mushrooms
1	cup short-grain brown rice
1	cup reduced-sodium beef broth
1	cup water
1/2	pound broccoli, cut into small florets
2	tablespoons sesame seeds
4	garlic cloves, minced
8	ounces boneless tuna fillet
1	tablespoon sesame oil
1/4	pound sugar snap peas
2	tablespoons jarred teriyaki sauce

1. Heat a medium saucepan over medium heat. Add the butter and mushrooms. Cook for 2 to 3 minutes, stirring often, or until the mushrooms are soft.

2. Add the rice and stir well. Add the broth and water. Bring to a boil. Cover and reduce to a simmer. Cook for 25 to 30 minutes, or until the rice is almost cooked through.

3. Layer the broccoli on top of the rice without stirring. Cover and cook for 5 minutes longer, or until the broccoli is tender-crisp and the rice is cooked through.

4. Place the sesame seeds and half the garlic on a sheet of wax paper. Roll the tuna in the mixture to coat.

5. Heat a small skillet over high heat. Add the oil and tuna. Cook for 2 minutes per side, or until the tuna is well seared but still pink and slightly translucent inside. Transfer to a cutting board. Thinly slice, top with the peas, and drizzle with the teriyaki sauce.

6. Serve immediately, separating the rice, broccoli, and tuna into small dishes, or cool before refrigerating in an airtight container.

PER SERVING: 411 calories, 22 g protein, 52 g carbohydrates, 6 g fiber, 11 g fat (2 g saturated), 460 mg sodium

PANZANELLA WITH SHRIMP

**Prep time: 10 minutes / Total time: 20 minutes /
Serves 4 (2 cups panzanella per serving)**

8	ounces country-style whole wheat bread or whole wheat baguette, cubed
1	pound tomatoes, chopped
1	small red onion, thinly sliced
1/4	cup red wine vinegar or malt vinegar
1	tablespoon olive oil
1/2	teaspoon paprika
1/2	pound medium shrimp
2	garlic cloves, minced
1	cup no-salt-added canned beans, such as garbanzo, navy, or cannellini, rinsed and drained
4	ounces fresh mozzarella cheese, cubed
1	cup basil, torn or thinly sliced

1. Place the bread, tomatoes, onion, and vinegar in a large bowl. Mix with your fingers, breaking up the bread and pressing the tomatoes to soak the bread cubes. Drizzle the oil over the mixture, sprinkle with the paprika, and toss again.

2. Heat a medium skillet over high heat. Coat with cooking spray and add the shrimp and garlic. Cook for 3 to 4 minutes, turning the shrimp occasionally, or until cooked through. Transfer to the bowl with the bread cubes, along with the beans, cheese, and basil. Toss and serve immediately.

PER SERVING: 411 calories, 25 g protein, 48 g carbohydrates, 6 g fiber, 12 g fat (4 g saturated), 560 mg sodium

{ **CHEF'S NOTE:** This recipe keeps well refrigerated overnight.

Dinner

If you're cooking dinner for your family, you'll find some favorites here that you can easily share. If you're on your own, just store the leftovers for quick meals later in the week. Each of the following recipes provides around 500 calories, with chewy proteins and hearty fiber-rich foods. Men, remember that you should add another 200 calories to each dinner.

BAKED ZITI

Prep time: 5 minutes / Total time: 35 minutes /
Serves 4 (1½ cups pasta and veggies per serving)

1	red bell pepper, seeded and chopped
2	carrots, grated
2	celery stalks, chopped
½	pound 7% lean ground turkey
1	teaspoon dried oregano
14	ounces whole grain or whole wheat ziti or penne, cooked according to package directions (note that this is half a box)
1	cup part-skim ricotta cheese
1½	cups jarred marinara sauce
1	cup grated part-skim mozzarella cheese

1. Preheat the oven to 400°F. Heat a large skillet over high heat. Coat with cooking spray and add the pepper, carrots, celery, turkey, and oregano. Cook for 1 minute without stirring to brown the turkey. Cook for 3 to 4 minutes longer, stirring occasionally, breaking up the turkey while you stir. Turn off the heat.

2. Add the pasta and ricotta and toss to coat. Transfer to an 8″ × 12″ casserole dish. Pour the marinara sauce over the pasta mixture and sprinkle with the mozzarella. Bake for 15 to 20 minutes, or until the cheese is bubbly and begins to brown. Cool for 5 minutes before serving.

PER SERVING: 496 calories, 41 g protein, 47 g carbohydrates, 8 g fiber, 16 g fat (6 g saturated), 764 mg sodium

NO-BOIL MANICOTTI

Prep time: 10 minutes / Total time: 35 minutes /
Serves 4 (1½ cups, including sauce and pasta, per serving)

2	large sweet potatoes
2	cups baby spinach, chopped
1	cup part-skim ricotta cheese
2	egg whites
2	tablespoons ground golden flaxseed
1	can (28 ounces) no-salt-added whole, peeled or diced tomatoes, pureed
20	fresh wonton wrappers (2″)
1	cup grated part-skim mozzarella cheese

1. Pierce each sweet potato twice with a fork. Wrap in a paper towel and place on a microwave-safe dish. Microwave on high for 4 minutes, or until soft to the touch. Remove the skin and mash the sweet potato until smooth.

2. Preheat the oven to 400°F. Place the spinach, sweet potato, ricotta, egg whites, and flaxseed in a medium bowl. Mix with a wooden spoon until well combined.

3. Spread half the tomato puree over the bottom of an 8″ × 12″ baking dish.

4. Spoon 2 tablespoons of the filling onto the center of 1 wonton wrapper. Fold 2 of the sides over to cover the filling. Place the stuffed wonton wrapper, seam side down, in the baking dish on top of the tomato puree.

5. Repeat with the remaining wonton wrappers. Spoon the remaining tomato puree on top and sprinkle with the mozzarella. Bake for 20 to 25 minutes, or until the cheese is bubbly and brown. Serve immediately.

PER SERVING: 511 calories, 27 g protein, 67 g carbohydrates, 13 g fat (7 g saturated), 51 mg cholesterol, 5 g fiber, 832 mg sodium

CHEF'S NOTE: Wonton wrappers can be found in most major grocery chains, usually in the refrigerated section of the produce aisle where they sell tofu.

PINEAPPLE-CHICKEN RICE BOWL

Prep time: 10 minutes / Total time: 20 minutes /
Serves 4 (1½ cups chicken and vegetable mixture, plus ½ cup rice, per serving)

1	cup uncooked short-grain brown rice
2	small boneless, skinless chicken breasts, cut into strips (about ½ pound)
2	tablespoons reduced-sodium soy sauce
2	teaspoons cornstarch
1	teaspoon packed light brown sugar
2	tablespoons sesame oil
1	pound collard greens, trimmed and thinly sliced
½	pound shiitake mushrooms, stems removed and thinly sliced
1	piece (1") fresh ginger, peeled and chopped
4	garlic cloves, minced
1	cup frozen edamame, rinsed under hot water
8	ounces fresh pineapple, cubed
1	cup reduced-sodium chicken or vegetable broth
1	tablespoon sesame seeds, toasted

1. Cook the rice according to package instructions. Set aside.

2. Toss the chicken in a large bowl with the soy sauce, cornstarch, and brown sugar.

3. Heat a large skillet over high heat. Add the sesame oil and then immediately add the chicken. Cook for 1 to 2 minutes, or until the chicken begins to brown. Add the collards, mushrooms, ginger, and garlic and cook for 3 to 4 minutes longer, stirring often. Add a few tablespoons of water if the mixture sticks.

4. Add the edamame, pineapple, and broth. Cover and then reduce to a simmer.

5. Cook for 1 to 2 minutes, or until half the liquid evaporates and a sauce has formed. Sprinkle with the sesame seeds and serve with the rice.

PER SERVING: 501 calories, 27 g protein, 68 g carbohydrates, 8 g fiber, 14 g fat (2 g saturated), 476 mg sodium

CHEF'S NOTE: You can substitute frozen peas for the edamame, if you prefer.

CASHEW EGG ROLLS

Prep time: 10 minutes / Total time: 30 minutes / Serves 4 (3 large egg rolls per serving)

2	tablespoons olive oil
1/3	pound lean ground turkey (7% fat)
2	carrots, peeled and shredded
4	heads Belgian endive or 1/2 head red cabbage, finely shredded
1	cup chopped shiitake mushrooms (about 6 medium mushrooms)
1/4	cup water
1/3	cup cashew pieces
4	teaspoons oyster sauce
12	square egg roll wrappers (7")

1. Preheat the oven to 400°F. Heat a large skillet over high heat and coat with cooking spray. Add 1 teaspoon of the oil. Add the turkey, carrots, endive or cabbage, and mushrooms. Cook for 7 to 8 minutes, stirring often while breaking up the meat with the back of a wooden spoon.

2. Add the water and scrape up any bits sticking to the bottom of the pan. Remove from the heat, then stir in the cashews and oyster sauce.

3. Place 1/4 cup water in a shallow bowl. Set out the egg roll wrappers on a clean countertop. Evenly divide the filling among the wrappers. Fold the 2 opposite corners in to touch, then fold in 1 of the other corners. Brush the remaining unfolded corner with water, then roll up the filling over the damp corner to close. Repeat.

4. Heat the remaining oil in a large oven-safe skillet over medium heat and add the egg rolls. Cook for 1 to 2 minutes, turning once, or until the wrappers brown. Slide the skillet into the oven and bake for 5 to 6 minutes, or until the filling is hot. Serve immediately.

PER SERVING: 484 calories, 19 g protein, 65 g carbohydrates, 4 g fiber, 16 g fat (2 g saturated), 763 mg sodium

CHEF'S NOTE: Because these egg rolls aren't deep-fried, they reheat nicely on a dry baking sheet in a 400°F oven or in a toaster oven. Just refrigerate overnight.

You can use almonds instead of the cashews, but cashews really make this dish.

BACON-AND-BROCCOLI BOW TIES

Prep time: 5 minutes / Total time: 15 minutes / Serves 4

1   jar (12 ounces) roasted red peppers

2   tablespoons red wine vinegar

¼   cup water

1   tablespoon olive oil

1   head broccoli, cut into small florets

3   slices nitrate-free turkey bacon, chopped

3   garlic cloves, minced

12   ounces whole grain pasta or brown rice pasta, cooked according to package directions

1   cup grated Parmesan cheese

1. Place the peppers (with juice), vinegar, and water in a blender or food processor. Blend until smooth.

2. Heat the oil in a large skillet over high heat. Add the broccoli, bacon, and garlic. Decrease the heat to medium and cook for 4 to 5 minutes, stirring often, or until the broccoli starts to soften.

3. Reduce the heat to low and add the roasted red-pepper sauce and cook for 2 to 3 minutes longer, or until the sauce starts to thicken. Toss in the pasta and cheese and serve immediately.

PER SERVING: 510 calories, 24 g protein, 79 g carbohydrates, 15 g fiber, 13 g fat (5 g saturated), 701 mg sodium

BALSAMIC CHICKEN AND PASTA

Prep time: 10 minutes / Total time: 20 minutes /
Serves 4 (2 cups pasta with chicken and veggies)

2	teaspoons extra-virgin olive oil
2	teaspoons whole wheat flour
1	bunch asparagus, trimmed and cut into 1" pieces
1/2	red onion, diced
1/4	teaspoon freshly ground black pepper
1/4	teaspoon crushed red-pepper flakes
1/4	teaspoon salt
1/4	cup white wine
1/2	cup balsamic vinegar
1	package (8 ounces) fresh whole wheat pasta, cooked according to package directions
1	pint cherry or grape tomatoes, cut in half
1	cup reduced-sodium chicken stock
1	head radicchio (about 10 ounces), thinly sliced
2	cooked chicken breasts, cubed
1	cup cubed fresh mozzarella cheese or bite-size mozzarella balls

1. Heat the oil in a large skillet over medium-high heat. Add the flour, asparagus, onion, black pepper, red-pepper flakes, and salt. Cook for 2 to 3 minutes, or until the onion is lightly browned.

2. Add the wine and vinegar. Cook for 1 to 2 minutes, scraping up any bits sticking to the bottom of the pan, or until the vegetables soften.

3. Add the pasta, along with the tomatoes and stock. Cook for 1 minute longer, or until the pasta is warm. Stir in the radicchio and chicken and top with the cheese. Serve immediately.

PER SERVING: 517 calories, 35 g protein, 63 g carbohydrates, 12 g fiber, 14 g fat (6 g saturated), 510 mg sodium

CHEF'S NOTE: You can substitute thinly sliced red cabbage for the radicchio, if you prefer.

SHEPHERD'S PIE

**Prep time: 10 minutes / Total time: 1 hour 15 minutes /
Serves 4 (2 cups, including filling and topping, per serving)**

4	medium white potatoes, such as russet, cubed (about 2 pounds)
½	cup milk
½	cup reduced-fat sour cream
1	tablespoon olive oil
½	pound lean ground turkey (7% fat)
1	small onion, peeled and chopped
1	tablespoon Worcestershire sauce
1	teaspoon chopped rosemary
1	teaspoon chili powder
¼	teaspoon salt
1	tablespoon whole wheat flour
2	carrots, chopped
2	tomatoes, chopped
2	egg whites
1	cup whole wheat bread crumbs
¼	cup grated Parmesan cheese

1. Place the potatoes in a large stockpot filled with cold water. Bring to a boil, then reduce to a simmer. Cook for 20 to 25 minutes, uncovered, or until the potatoes are tender when pierced with a fork. Drain. Transfer one-quarter of the potatoes to a large bowl and drizzle with ¼ cup of the milk and ¼ cup of the sour cream.

2. Beat on low speed with an electric mixer and repeat, slowly adding the remaining ¼ cup milk and ¼ cup sour cream, until the potatoes are completely mashed together with the sour cream and milk.

3. Preheat the oven to 350°F. Heat the oil in a large skillet over medium heat. Add the turkey, onion, Worcestershire sauce, rosemary, chili powder, and salt and cook for 3 to 4 minutes, breaking up the turkey with the back of a wooden spoon.

4. Add the flour and cook for 1 minute, stirring often, or until the flour starts to coat the bottom of the pan.

5. Stir in the carrots and tomatoes and cook for 2 to 3 minutes longer.

6. Transfer to an 8" × 12" casserole dish. Stir the egg whites into the potatoes. Spoon them over the meat mixture and sprinkle with the bread crumbs and cheese. Baked for 40 to 45 minutes, uncovered, or until the topping is brown and puffed.

PER SERVING: 505 calories, 27 g protein, 70 g carbohydrates, 7 g fiber, 13 g fat (5 g saturated), 529 mg sodium

SPAGHETTI AND MEATBALLS

**Prep time: 5 minutes / Total time: 45 minutes /
Serves 4 (5 meatballs plus 1½ cups pasta per serving)**

6	ounces whole wheat bread (about 3 slices sandwich bread)
½	cup fat-free milk
½	pound lean ground turkey (7% fat)
5	ounces broccoli rabe, chopped
2	garlic cloves, minced
1	egg
1	teaspoon dried oregano
1	tablespoon olive oil
½	cup white wine
1	can (28 ounces) chopped tomatoes
½	red onion, chopped
¼	teaspoon salt
½	cup grated Parmesan cheese
8	ounces whole wheat angel-hair pasta, cooked according to package directions

1. Place the bread and milk in a large bowl. Mix well until the bread absorbs the milk, breaking up the bread with your fingers.

2. Add the turkey, broccoli rabe, garlic, egg, and oregano. Mix well until the turkey and bread are well incorporated. Form the turkey into 20 meatballs and place on a sheet of wax paper.

3. Heat the oil in a large skillet over medium-high heat. Carefully add the meatballs and cook for 1 to 2 minutes, or until the meatballs begin to brown, then turn them.

4. Add the wine and cook for 1 to 2 minutes, or until the wine decreases by half.

5. Add the tomatoes (with juice), onion, and salt. Reduce the heat to low. Cook for 20 to 25 minutes, covered, or until the meatballs are cooked through. Serve immediately with the cheese and pasta.

PER SERVING: 505 calories, 32 g protein, 64 g carbohydrates, 11 g fiber, 12 g fat (3 g saturated), 490 mg sodium

CHEF'S NOTE: You can substitute collard greens for the broccoli rabe, if you prefer.

162

CHICKEN-PESTO PARMESAN

Prep time: 5 minutes / **Total time:** 25 minutes /
Serves 4 (1 chicken cutlet, $1/2$ cup cooked pasta tossed in sauce,
and $1/2$ cup broccoli per serving)

1	cup packed basil
3	tablespoons pine nuts
2	garlic cloves, cut in half
1	egg
1	cup seasoned whole wheat bread crumbs
4	thinly sliced raw chicken cutlets (about 1 pound)
1	tablespoon extra-virgin olive oil
1	can (28 ounces) unsalted whole, peeled tomatoes
4	cups fresh broccoli florets
$1/2$	cup grated Parmesan cheese
4	ounces whole wheat angel-hair pasta, cooked according to package directions

1. Preheat the oven to 400°F. Place the basil, pine nuts, and garlic in a food processor and pulse 5 or 6 times, or until the leaves are chopped. With the motor running, add the egg until a thick sauce forms. Transfer the mixture to a shallow bowl.

2. Place the bread crumbs on a sheet of wax paper. Dip both sides of the chicken into the pesto mixture and then press into the bread crumbs.

3. Heat the oil in a large oven-safe skillet over medium heat. Add the chicken and cook for 4 to 5 minutes, turning once, or until the bread crumbs are golden.

4. Spoon the canned tomatoes around the chicken and arrange the broccoli florets around the outside edges of the skillet. Sprinkle the cheese over the chicken.

5. Slide the skillet into the oven and bake for 10 to 15 minutes, or until the cheese is golden and the broccoli is tender-crisp. Serve immediately with the pasta.

PER SERVING: 509 calories, 35 g protein, 58 g carbohydrates, 10 g fiber, 13 g fat (2 g saturated), 628 mg sodium

ORANGE-SESAME CHICKEN

Prep time: 10 minutes / Total time: 20 minutes /
Serves 4 (1½ cups orange-sesame chicken and ½ cup cooked rice per serving)

¾   cup orange juice

¼   cup apple cider
     vinegar

2   tablespoons
     reduced-sodium
     soy sauce

1   tablespoon packed
     light brown sugar

2   teaspoons
     cornstarch

2   tablespoons
     sesame oil

3   large boneless,
     skinless chicken
     breasts, thinly sliced
     (about 1½ pounds)

2   garlic cloves

1   piece (1") ginger,
     chopped

1   teaspoon red-
     pepper flakes

4   celery stalks,
     thinly sliced

4   carrots, peeled and
     thinly sliced

2   cups frozen peas,
     rinsed under hot
     running water

2   tablespoons sesame
     seeds, toasted

2   cups cooked
     short-grain
     brown rice

1. Place the juice, vinegar, soy sauce, brown sugar, and cornstarch in a small bowl and whisk until smooth.

2. Heat a large skillet over high heat. Add 1 tablespoon of the oil, the chicken, garlic, ginger, and red-pepper flakes. Cook for 4 to 5 minutes, or until the chicken begins to brown. Transfer to a plate.

3. Add the celery, carrots, and remaining 1 tablespoon oil. Cook for 2 to 3 minutes, or until the celery begins to soften.

4. Return the chicken to the pan, along with the peas. Reduce the heat to low and add the juice mixture. Cook for 2 to 3 minutes longer, scraping up any bits of chicken sticking to the bottom of the pan. Sprinkle with the sesame seeds and serve immediately with the rice.

PER SERVING: 532 calories, 45 g protein, 53 g carbohydrates, 8 g fiber, 15 g fat (2 g saturated), 625 mg sodium

CASHEW CHICKEN

Prep time: 5 minutes / Total time: 20 minutes /
Serves 4 (2 ounces noodles plus 2 cups vegetables and chicken per serving)

3	tablespoons oyster sauce
3	tablespoons water
2	teaspoons cornstarch
2	teaspoons rice vinegar
2	garlic cloves, minced
1	teaspoon sugar
1	pound asparagus, trimmed and cut into thirds
1/2	pound Brussels sprouts, quartered
6	ounces shiitake mushrooms, sliced (discard stems)
1	small red onion, diced
2	boneless, skinless chicken breasts, cut into 1/2"-thick chunks (about 1 pound)
1/2	cup cashew pieces
8	ounces soba noodles, cooked according to package directions

1. Place the oyster sauce, water, cornstarch, vinegar, garlic, and sugar in a small bowl. Whisk until smooth.

2. Heat a large skillet over high heat. Add the asparagus, Brussels sprouts, mushrooms, and onion. Cook for 2 to 3 minutes, stirring often, or until the onion starts to soften.

3. Add the chicken and cook for 2 to 3 minutes longer, or until the outside of the chicken turns white.

4. Add the sauce and cover. Reduce the heat to low and cook for 3 to 4 minutes, or until the sauce thickens and the chicken is cooked through. Sprinkle with the cashews and serve immediately with the noodles.

PER SERVING: 513 calories, 28 g protein, 72 g carbohydrates, 9 g fiber, 14 g fat (3 g saturated), 595 mg sodium

CHEF'S NOTE: You can substitute red cabbage for the Brussels sprouts, if you prefer.

STUFFED-PEPPER BAKE

Prep time: 5 minutes / Total time: 30 minutes /
Serves 4 (1 stuffed pepper with 2 cups filling per serving)

4	poblanos or 4 green or red bell peppers
1	tablespoon olive oil
$\frac{1}{2}$	pound lean ground turkey (7% fat)
1	small zucchini, diced
$\frac{1}{2}$	red onion
1	tablespoon fresh thyme
1	teaspoon paprika
$\frac{1}{4}$	teaspoon salt
2	cups baby spinach leaves, packed
2	tablespoons raisins
1	cup grated pepper Jack or sharp Cheddar cheese

1. Place the peppers directly on a gas burner on low heat. Roast for 15 to 20 minutes. Turn often, until the skins are well charred. Transfer to a medium bowl and cover tightly with plastic wrap.

2. Heat a large skillet over high heat and add the oil. Add the turkey, zucchini, onion, thyme, paprika, and salt. Cook for 4 to 5 minutes, breaking up the turkey as you stir.

3. Add the spinach and raisins and cook for 1 minute longer, or until the spinach wilts. Turn off the heat.

4. Remove the plastic wrap from the peppers and peel off the charred skin. Remove the stems and discard the seeds.

5. Place the peppers in an 8" × 12" baking dish and stuff them with the spinach mixture. Sprinkle the cheese over the peppers and bake for 20 to 25 minutes, uncovered, or until the cheese melts and the filling is hot. Serve immediately.

PER SERVING: 500 calories, 21 g protein, 55 g carbohydrates, 6 g fiber, 14 g fat (5 g saturated), 580 mg sodium

HUNGARIAN BEEF STEW

Prep time: 10 minutes / Total time: 1 hour 45 minutes /
Serves 4 (2 cups stew per serving)

1	tablespoon whole wheat flour
1	tablespoon paprika
1	teaspoon hot paprika or cayenne
1	pound lean beef stew, trimmed of excess fat
¼	teaspoon salt
2	teaspoons olive oil
¼	cup tomato paste
¼	cup white wine
3	cups reduced-sodium beef broth
4	medium carrots, peeled and cut into 1" pieces
3	medium white potatoes, such as Yukon gold, cubed (about ¾ pound)
1	bag (10 ounces) frozen green peas, defrosted

1. Place the flour and both types of paprika, or the paprika and cayenne, on a sheet of wax paper. Mix the flour into the paprika, using your fingertips. Sprinkle the beef with the salt and then roll it in the paprika mixture. Shake off any excess flour and set the beef on a plate.

2. Heat a large stockpot over medium heat. Add the oil and beef. Cook for 4 to 5 minutes, turning occasionally, or until the beef is lightly browned.

3. Add the tomato paste and cook another minute, or until the paste becomes fragrant.

4. Add the wine, broth, carrots, and potatoes. Cover and cook for about 1½ hours, stirring occasionally, or until the beef is very tender and the liquid has formed a thick sauce. Stir in the peas before serving.

PER SERVING: 501 calories, 44 g protein, 39 g carbohydrates, 8 g fiber, 15 g fat (5 g saturated), 716 mg sodium

MOIST MEAT LOAF WITH SWEET POTATO MASH

Prep time: 5 minutes / Total time: 50 minutes /
Serves 4 (2 slices meat loaf and 1½ cups mashed potatoes per serving)

2	slices whole wheat bread, cubed
1	cup grated zucchini
¼	cup fat-free milk
1	egg
3	garlic cloves
2	tablespoons Worcestershire sauce
¼	cup chopped basil or parsley
1	pound dark-meat ground turkey
3	tablespoons ketchup or barbecue sauce
5	medium sweet potatoes, peeled and cubed (about 1½ pounds)
1	cup reduced-fat sour cream
1	tablespoon hot sauce
4	scallions, thinly sliced

1. Preheat the oven to 350°F. Place the bread, zucchini, milk, egg, garlic, Worcestershire sauce, and basil or parsley in a large bowl. Break up the bread pieces with your fingers while tossing them to moisten. Add the turkey and mix well.

2. Transfer to a loaf pan, spread ketchup or barbecue sauce over the top with a rubber spatula and bake for 45 to 50 minutes, or until the meat is cooked through.

3. Place the sweet potatoes in a large stockpot and cover with cold water. Bring to a boil, then reduce to a steady simmer. Cook for 15 to 20 minutes, or until the potatoes are tender when pressed with a fork. Drain and transfer to a large bowl.

4. Gradually beat in the sour cream with an electric mixer on low speed. Add the hot sauce and scallions and serve immediately with the meat loaf.

PER SERVING: 508 calories, 32 g protein, 68 g carbohydrates, 9 g fiber, 12 g fat (4 g saturated), 472 mg sodium

HONEY-GLAZED PORK LOIN WITH GARLIC MASHED POTATOES

Prep time: 5 minutes / Total time: 1 hour /
Serves 4 (6 ounces pork, 1 cup mashed potatoes, and 1 cup broccoli per serving)

½ cup pomegranate or apple juice

2 tablespoons honey

1 tablespoon reduced-sodium soy sauce

4 garlic cloves, minced

1½ pounds pork tenderloin, trimmed of excess fat

¼ teaspoon cayenne

2 tablespoons olive oil

4 small white potatoes, such as Yukon gold (about 1½ pounds)

½ cup reduced-fat sour cream

¼ cup parsley, chopped

¼ teaspoon salt

4 cups broccoli florets, steamed

1. Preheat the oven to 400°F. Place the juice, honey, soy sauce, and half the garlic in a small bowl. Stir to combine. Sprinkle the pork with the cayenne.

2. Heat a medium skillet over high heat. Add 1 tablespoon of the oil. Add the pork and cook for 3 to 4 minutes, or until the pork is browned. Turn the meat and cook for 4 minutes longer. Turn off the heat. Pour the juice mixture over the pork and transfer to the oven.

3. Bake the pork for 25 to 30 minutes, or until no longer translucent when cut with a knife in the center but still slightly pink. Transfer to a cutting board.

4. Place the skillet back on the burner and cook the juice for 1 to 2 minutes, or until a thick glaze forms. Set aside off the heat.

5. Place the potatoes in a medium stockpot and fill with cold water. Bring to a boil over high heat and cook for 20 to 25 minutes, or until fork-tender. Drain and return the potatoes to the stockpot.

6. Add the sour cream, parsley, salt, and remaining 1 tablespoon oil and remaining garlic. Mash with an electric mixer or a handheld masher until smooth.

7. Slice the pork and pour the glaze over the slices. Serve with the mashed potatoes and broccoli.

PER SERVING: 481 calories, 42 g protein, 46 g carbohydrates, 7 g fiber, 15 g fat (5 g saturated), 560 mg sodium

FISH AND CHIPS

Prep time: 5 minutes / Total time: 30 minutes /
Serves 4 (3 ounces fish, 4 ounces fries, and $\frac{1}{2}$ cup veggies per serving)

1	pound frozen sweet potato fries
4	cups high-fiber cereal flakes
$\frac{1}{4}$	cup white whole wheat flour or whole wheat pastry flour
3	egg whites
12	ounces tilapia fillet, cut into strips
$\frac{1}{4}$	teaspoon salt
$\frac{1}{4}$	teaspoon paprika
1	tablespoon olive oil
1	pound asparagus, trimmed and cut into thirds
$\frac{1}{4}$	cup malt vinegar

1. Preheat the oven to 400°F. Spread out the fries on an ungreased baking sheet and bake according to package directions.

2. Place the cereal in a food processor and pulse until fine crumbs form. Spread out the crumbs on a sheet of wax paper, along with the flour.

3. Place the egg whites in a shallow bowl. Sprinkle the fish with the salt and paprika, then dip into the egg whites. Press both sides into the cereal mixture.

4. Heat a large skillet over high heat. Add the oil and fish strips. Cook for 2 minutes, or until the coating starts to brown. Turn the fish and scatter the asparagus around the fish.

5. Slide the skillet into the oven along with the fries and bake for 5 to 6 minutes, or until the fish is cooked through. Serve the fish and asparagus with the fries, along with the malt vinegar for dipping.

PER SERVING: 484 calories, 27 g protein, 59 g carbohydrates, 11 g fiber, 15 g fat (2 g saturated), 506 mg sodium

FISH IN A PACKET
WITH HOT BUTTERED RICE

Prep time: 5 minutes / Total time: 45 minutes /
Serves 4 (1 piece fish with $1/2$ cup sauce and 1 cup rice per serving)

1	tablespoon canola oil
1	tablespoon unsalted butter
2	garlic cloves, minced
$1/4$	cup chopped parsley
2	cups short-grain brown rice
4	cups water
2	large oranges, sectioned
1	pound tomatoes, diced (about 4 medium plum tomatoes)
1	cup jarred Peppadew peppers, thinly sliced
$1/2$	red onion, minced
	Zest and juice of 1 lemon
$1/2$	teaspoon salt
1	pound boneless, skinless cod fillets

1. Warm the oil and butter in a medium saucepan. Add the garlic and parsley and cook for 1 minute, stirring often.

2. Add the rice and stir until the grains are evenly coated in the oil. Add the water and bring to a boil. Cover and reduce to a simmer and cook for 25 to 30 minutes, or until the grains are soft.

3. Preheat the oven to 400°F. Toss the oranges, tomatoes, peppers, onion, lemon zest and juice, and $1/4$ teaspoon of the salt in a large bowl.

4. Set out four 12"-long sheets of aluminum foil. Place 1 fish fillet on each sheet and sprinkle with the remaining $1/4$ teaspoon salt. Evenly distribute the orange mixture over the fillets and fold the foil, crimping the edges to make packets. Transfer to a baking sheet and bake for 10 to 15 minutes, or until the fish is cooked through. Serve immediately with the rice.

PER SERVING: 511 calories, 26 g protein, 68 g carbohydrates, 7 g fiber, 12 g fat (3 g saturated), 426 mg sodium

ORANGE-SOY SALMON

Prep time: 5 minutes / Total time: 20 minutes /
Serves 4 (1 piece salmon, 1 cup brown rice, and 1 cup vegetables per serving)

4	oranges, zested and juiced
2	star anise pods
1	tablespoon reduced-sodium soy sauce
1	teaspoon sugar
2	teaspoons sesame oil
1	red or orange bell pepper, seeded and thinly sliced
1	yellow bell pepper, seeded and thinly sliced
1	small head radicchio (about 1 pound), thinly sliced
¼	teaspoon salt
4	boneless raw salmon fillets (4 ounces), skin on
5	cups brown rice, cooked according to package directions

1. Place the orange zest and juice, anise pods, soy sauce, and sugar in a small saucepan. Place over medium heat and cook for 2 to 3 minutes, or until the liquid decreases by one-third, stirring once or twice. Set aside.

2. Preheat the oven to 400°F. Heat a large skillet over medium-high heat. Coat with cooking spray. Add the oil and peppers and cook for 3 to 4 minutes, or until the peppers start to soften. Turn off the heat and, with a spoon, spread out the peppers so that they form an even layer.

3. Arrange the radicchio on top of the peppers and sprinkle with the salt. Place the salmon on top of the radicchio, skin side down.

4. Transfer the skillet to the oven and bake for 10 to 12 minutes, or until the salmon is almost cooked through and no longer translucent. Remove the star anise from the reserved orange glaze and drizzle over the salmon. Serve immediately with the brown rice.

PER SERVING: 501 calories, 27 g protein, 69 g carbohydrates, 8 g fiber, 13 g fat (1 g saturated), 493 mg sodium

CHEF'S NOTE: Cooked short-grain brown rice keeps extremely well in the fridge in an airtight container. Just add 1 tablespoon water before reheating in a covered saucepan over low heat for 2 minutes, or covered in the microwave for 30 seconds.

You can substitute a cinnamon stick for the star anise pods, if you prefer.

CARIBBEAN TILAPIA WITH PLANTAINS

Prep time: 5 minutes / Total time: 25 minutes /
Serves 4 (one 4-ounce piece of fish, 1 cup salsa, and 1 cup plantains per serving)

6	ounces pineapple chunks, chopped
$\frac{1}{2}$	cup fresh cilantro, chopped
1	small red onion, chopped
1	seeded habanero chile pepper or $\frac{1}{2}$ red bell pepper, chopped
1	lime, juiced
$\frac{1}{2}$	teaspoon salt
$\frac{1}{2}$	cup fine cornmeal
$\frac{1}{3}$	cup unsweetened coconut
1	egg
1	pound tilapia fish fillets
4	teaspoons canola oil
3	very ripe plantains with black skins, peeled and cut into 1" chunks

1. Place the pineapple, cilantro, onion, pepper, lime juice, and $\frac{1}{4}$ teaspoon of the salt in a large bowl. Toss and set aside.

2. Place the cornmeal and coconut on a sheet of wax paper and mix with your fingertips.

3. Place the egg in a shallow bowl. Sprinkle the fish with the remaining $\frac{1}{4}$ teaspoon salt. Dip the flesh side of the fish in the egg and then press only the flesh side into the coconut mixture.

4. Heat 2 teaspoons of the oil in a large skillet over medium heat. Add the plantains and cook for 5 to 10 minutes, turning occasionally, or until a golden crust forms.

5. In another large skillet, heat the remaining 2 teaspoons oil over medium heat. Add the fish, coconut coating down, and cook for 6 to 8 minutes, turning once, or until the fish flakes off when a fork is pressed against it. Serve the fish immediately with plantains and reserved salsa.

PER SERVING: 484 calories, 28 g protein, 68 g carbohydrates, 7 g fiber, 14 g fat (5 g saturated), 380 mg sodium

SHRIMP SCAMPI LINGUINE

**Prep time: 5 minutes / Total time: 20 minutes /
Serves 4 (2$\frac{1}{2}$ ounces pasta and 1$\frac{1}{2}$ cups topping per serving)**

9	ounces fresh whole wheat linguine
1	tablespoon extra-virgin olive oil
4	garlic cloves, minced
$\frac{1}{2}$	teaspoon red-pepper flakes
1	pound medium shrimp, peeled and deveined
1	pint cherry tomatoes, cut in half
$\frac{1}{2}$	cup dry white wine
	Juice of 1 lemon
$\frac{1}{2}$	teaspoon salt
3	cups packed baby spinach leaves
$\frac{1}{4}$	cup finely chopped parsley leaves
$\frac{1}{2}$	cup grated Parmesan cheese

1. Cook the pasta according to package directions. Drain the pasta and set aside.

2. Heat a large skillet over medium heat. Add the oil, garlic, and red-pepper flakes and cook for 1 minute, or until the garlic starts to brown.

3. Toss in the shrimp and cook for 2 minutes longer, or until the shrimp start to turn pink.

4. Add the tomatoes, wine, lemon juice, and salt. Cook 1 minute longer, or until the tomatoes start to soften and the liquid reduces.

5. Toss in the reserved pasta, the spinach, and parsley. Toss to coat and serve with the cheese.

PER SERVING: 483 calories, 38 g protein, 50 g carbohydrates, 11 g fiber, 13 g fat (3 g saturated), 665 mg sodium

PEANUT NOODLES

Prep time: 10 minutes / Total time: 25 minutes / Serves 4 (2 cups noodles per serving)

12	ounces raw soba noodles
1½	cups reduced-fat coconut milk
¼	cup creamy peanut butter
1	tablespoon reduced-sodium soy sauce
1	teaspoon hot sauce, such as Tabasco or sriracha
1	pound medium shrimp, shelled and deveined
3	carrots, thinly sliced
3	celery stalks, thinly sliced
2	garlic cloves, chopped
1	piece (1") ginger, peeled and chopped
2	cups baby spinach

1. Cook the noodles according to package directions. Drain and set aside.

2. Whisk the coconut milk, peanut butter, soy sauce, and hot sauce in a medium bowl.

3. Heat a large skillet over medium heat. Coat with cooking spray and add the shrimp, carrots, celery, garlic, and ginger.

4. Cook for 4 to 5 minutes, or until the vegetables start to soften and the shrimp begin to brown. Add a few tablespoons of water if the vegetables start to stick. Add the spinach and cook for 1 minute longer, or until it wilts.

5. Add the reserved noodles and peanut sauce. Toss to combine and serve immediately.

PER SERVING: 514 calories, 35 g protein, 64 g carbohydrates, 1 g fiber, 13 g fat (5 g saturated), 484 mg sodium

MUSSELS WITH SPICY BROTH AND STEAK FRIES

Prep time: 10 minutes / Total time: 30 minutes / Serves 4 (1/2 pound mussels plus 1/2 cup sauce, 1/2 cup veggies, and 1 cup potato wedges per serving)

6	medium red potatoes, cut into 1"-thick wedges (about 2 1/2 pounds)
2	tablespoons olive oil
5	garlic cloves, minced
1/4	cup Italian parsley, packed
1/2	teaspoon hot paprika
1/4	teaspoon coarsely ground black pepper
1/4	teaspoon salt
2	pounds mussels, such as blue or Prince Edward Island
1	pound tomatoes (about 4 medium), chopped
1	bunch watercress (about 3 ounces), trimmed
1/2	cup dry white wine
2	Belgian endive bulbs (about 6 ounces), trimmed and quartered

1. Place the potatoes in a stockpot filled with cold water. Bring to a boil over high heat, then reduce to a simmer. Cook for 10 to 12 minutes, or until the potatoes are soft when pierced with a fork. Drain.

2. Heat 1 tablespoon of the oil in a large skillet. Add the potatoes and cook for 5 to 6 minutes, turning once or twice, or until the potatoes are brown and crisp. Sprinkle with half the garlic, the parsley, paprika, pepper, and salt. Cook for 1 minute longer, or until the garlic is fragrant. Turn off the heat and set aside the potatoes.

3. Place the mussels in a strainer in the sink and run cold running water over them. Remove the threadlike piece (also called the beard) that might be hanging from the hinge side of the shell.

4. Heat a large stockpot over medium heat. Add the remaining 1 tablespoon oil and remaining garlic. Cook for 1 minute, or until the garlic is fragrant and starts to turn golden.

5. Add the tomatoes and watercress and cook for 2 minutes longer, stirring once or twice, or until the tomatoes start to give off their liquid.

6. Add the wine, mussels, and endive. Cover tightly and cook for 7 to 9 minutes, or until the mussels are open and the meat is firm to the touch. Discard any shells that didn't open and serve the remaining mussels and sauce immediately with the reserved fries.

PER SERVING: 520 calories, 34 g protein, 62 g carbohydrates, 8 g fiber, 12 g fat (2 g saturated), 758 mg sodium

CHEF'S NOTE: You can substitute spinach for the watercress here, if you prefer.

Snacks and Desserts

I know that the secret to staying on a diet is not feeling as if you're dieting. So to give you as much flexibility as possible, I've included some scrumptious snack and dessert recipes here. On most days, you should limit yourself to either a snack or dessert of about 200 calories. But once in a while, you might really want both. On those days, try to stick to the 100-calorie options opposite (or have a "lunch" option for dinner) so that you stay in the 1,500-calorie range for the day (1,800 calories for men).

200-CALORIE SNACKS AND DESSERTS

100-CALORIE SNACKS AND DESSERTS

BLACK BEAN HUMMUS WITH TOASTED PITA

Prep time: 5 minutes / Total time: 10 minutes /
Serves 4 (¼ heaping cup hummus with 4 wedges pita per serving)

1	cup no-salt-added canned black beans (rinsed and drained)
1	lime, juiced
2	tablespoons light mayonnaise
2	garlic cloves, minced
¼	teaspoon salt
3	whole wheat pitas (6" diameter), cut into 4 wedges

Place the beans, lime juice, mayonnaise, garlic, and salt in a food processor. Blend until smooth and serve immediately with the pita wedges.

PER SERVING: 218 calories, 4 g protein, 34 g carbohydrates, 3 g fiber, 7 g fat (0 g saturated), 99 mg sodium

SWEET POTATO CHIPS

Prep time: 5 minutes / Total time: 10 minutes / Serves 4 (2 cups per serving)

3	sweet potatoes, skins on (about 1½ pounds)
3	tablespoons finely grated Parmesan cheese
¼	teaspoon cayenne
1	teaspoon lemon pepper
1	teaspoon garlic powder
1	teaspoon mild chili powder
1	tablespoon olive oil

1. Preheat the oven to 400°F. Coat 3 baking sheets with cooking spray. Thinly slice the sweet potatoes with a Japanese mandoline or plastic vegetable cutter.

2. Place the cheese, cayenne, lemon pepper, garlic powder, and chili powder in a small bowl and mix well.

3. Working in 3 batches, add 1 teaspoon of the oil to a large skillet over high heat. Add one-third of the potatoes and cook for 2 to 3 minutes, stirring often, or until the potatoes turn a shade darker. Sprinkle with one-third of the spice mix, then transfer to a baking sheet and spread out. Repeat with the remaining 2 batches.

4. Bake the chips for 8 to 10 minutes, or until perfectly crisp. Cool directly on the baking sheets and then serve immediately. Wrap loosely in aluminum foil to store.

PER SERVING: 197 calories, 4 g protein, 34 g carbohydrates, 5 g fiber, 4 g fat (1 g saturated), 125 mg sodium

CHEF'S NOTE: Storing the chips in aluminum foil keeps them crisp.

CORN MUFFINS
WITH COLBY AND JALAPEÑO

Prep time: 10 minutes / Total time: 20 minutes /
Makes 10 muffins (1 muffin per serving)

1	box (8.5 ounces) corn muffin mix
1/3	cup ground flaxseed
1/2	cup shredded low-fat Colby or Cheddar cheese
1/3	cup fat-free milk
2	jalapeño chile peppers, seeded and diced
1	egg
2	egg whites

1. Preheat the oven to 400°F. Coat a 12-cup muffin pan with cooking spray or line with muffin papers. Place the corn muffin mix and flaxseed in a large bowl. Stir with a wooden spoon until combined.

2. With the spoon, make a well in the center. Add the cheese, milk, peppers, egg, and egg whites. Starting from the center of the well, mix the well ingredients into the cheese, gradually combining with about 15 turns, or until a lumpy batter forms. Do not overmix or there will be dry spots.

3. Spoon the batter into 10 of the muffin cups, filling each two-thirds of the way. Bake for 8 to 10 minutes, or until the center of a muffin springs back to the touch when pressed. Remove the muffins from the pan and serve immediately. Or cool completely on a wire rack before storing in an airtight container for up to 3 days.

PER SERVING: 195 calories, 6 g protein, 19 g carbohydrates, 3 g fiber, 3 g fat (1 g saturated), 353 mg sodium

RASPBERRY-FILLED OAT BARS

Prep time: 10 minutes / Total time: 40 minutes /
Makes 10 bars (one 2" × 2" bar per serving)

½ cup light brown sugar, packed

¼ cup canola oil

2 tablespoons fat-free milk

1 egg

1 teaspoon vanilla extract

1¼ cups old-fashioned oats

1 cup white whole wheat flour or whole wheat pastry flour

½ teaspoon baking soda

½ teaspoon baking powder

2 tablespoons ground flaxseed

1 teaspoon ground cinnamon

⅛ teaspoon cayenne

¼ cup raspberry jam

1 apple, cored and sliced

1. Preheat the oven to 350°F. Place the brown sugar, oil, milk, egg, and vanilla extract in a large bowl. Stir until well combined.

2. Mix in the oats, flour, baking soda, baking powder, flaxseed, cinnamon, and cayenne. Stir until well combined.

3. Spoon half the batter into a 1-pound loaf pan or two ½-pound loaf pans. Spoon on the raspberry jam and apple. Top with the remaining batter.

4. Bake for 20 to 25 minutes, or until the top is firm to the touch. Cool completely in the pan.

5. Slice into 10 squares and serve. Or place in an airtight container and store on the countertop for up to 4 days.

PER SERVING: 218 calories, 4 g protein, 34 g carbohydrates, 3 g fiber, 7 g fat (0 g saturated), 99 mg sodium

CHEF'S NOTE: Avoid stone-ground whole wheat flour. White whole wheat and whole wheat pastry flour are more tender types of whole wheat flour. King Arthur and Arrowhead Mills, among other brands, make these types of flour.

CARAMEL APPLE CAKE

Prep time: 5 minutes / **Total time:** 1 hour 10 minutes /
Serves 12 (one 1" × 5" piece per serving)

1 tablespoon whole wheat flour

1 box (18 ounces) cake mix, yellow or white

⅓ cup ground flaxseed

1 teaspoon ground cinnamon

Pinch of cayenne

⅔ cup water

½ cup fat-free plain yogurt

3 egg whites

1 tablespoon canola oil

2 apples, cored, peeled, and thinly sliced

1 tablespoon grated fresh ginger

½ cup fat-free caramel sauce

1. Preheat the oven to 350°F. Coat a fluted tube pan with cooking spray and sprinkle with the flour. Set aside.

2. Place the cake mix in a large bowl with the flaxseed, cinnamon, and cayenne. Whisk to combine.

3. Add the water, yogurt, egg whites, and oil. Beat with an electric mixer on low speed for about 1 minute, or until a smooth, thick batter forms.

4. Spoon half the batter into the cake pan. Arrange the apple slices over the batter. Scatter the ginger on top, then drizzle with the caramel sauce.

5. Spoon the remaining batter on top and bake for 1 hour, or until the cake springs back when pressed. Cool for 2 to 3 minutes in the pan, then turn out on a wire rack to cool completely. Store in an airtight container on the countertop for up to 3 days or freeze, tightly wrapped, for up to 3 months.

PER SERVING: 225 calories, 2 g protein, 43 g carbohydrates, 3 g fiber, 1 g fat (0 g saturated), 296 mg sodium

CHEF'S NOTE: This cake gets more moist as it sits, so it's best to make it a day before you plan to serve.

COFFEE BANANAS FOSTER

Prep time: 5 minutes / Total time: 10 minutes /
Serves 4 (½ cup coffee frozen yogurt and ⅓ cup topping per serving)

2	teaspoons unsalted butter
2	bananas, cut into 1" chunks (about 12 ounces)
1	teaspoon ground cinnamon
	Pinch of cayenne
2	teaspoons packed light brown sugar
1	shot almond-flavored liqueur
¼	cup brewed coffee, cold or hot
2	cups fat-free coffee frozen yogurt

1. Heat a medium skillet over medium-high heat. Coat with cooking spray and add the butter. Once the butter has melted and started to bubble, add the bananas. Sprinkle the cinnamon, cayenne, and brown sugar over the bananas. Reduce the heat to medium and continue to cook for 2 to 3 minutes, turning occasionally, or until the bananas brown and the spices become fragrant.

2. Carefully pour in the liqueur and coffee. Cook for 1 minute longer, or until the liquid reduces slightly.

3. Place ½ cup of the frozen yogurt in each of 4 small bowls. Distribute the topping among the bowls and serve immediately.

PER SERVING: 229 calories, 5 g protein, 46 g carbohydrates, 2 g fiber, 2 g fat (0 g saturated), 67 mg sodium

CHEF'S NOTE: You can substitute coffee-flavored liqueur for the almond-flavored liqueur, if you prefer.

TANGY BLUE CHEESE DIP WITH VEGGIES

Prep time: 5 minutes / Total time: 10 minutes / Serves 4 (1 scant ¼ cup dip and ¼ pound vegetables per serving)

⅓ cup crumbled blue cheese

⅓ cup 0% fat plain Greek yogurt

2 tablespoons fat-free milk

1 tablespoon hot sauce

¼ teaspoon freshly ground black pepper

½ pound celery, cut into matchsticks

½ pound carrots, peeled and cut into matchsticks

1. Place the cheese in a large bowl. Mash with a wooden spoon, breaking up the crumbles.

2. Add the yogurt, milk, hot sauce, and pepper, mashing to combine. Serve immediately with the vegetable sticks.

PER SERVING: 96 calories, 5 g protein, 11 g carbohydrates, 3 g fiber, 3 g fat (2 g saturated), 392 mg sodium

ALMOND BUTTER CARAMEL CORN

Prep time: 5 minutes / Total time: 30 minutes /
Serves 8 (1 cup caramel corn per serving)

8	cups air-popped corn
4	tablespoons molasses
4	tablespoons almond butter

1. Preheat the oven to 300°F. Cover a baking sheet with aluminum foil and coat with cooking spray.

2. Place the popcorn in a large bowl and set out 2 large spoons.

3. Place the molasses and almond butter in a small saucepan and place over low heat. Cook for 1 to 2 minutes, stirring constantly, or until the almond butter has melted and the mixture is liquid.

4. Working quickly before the mixture cools, drizzle it over the popcorn and toss with the spoons.

5. Spread out the popcorn mixture on the cookie sheets and bake for 15 to 20 minutes, or until the surface of the corn is dry. Cool on the baking sheets, then serve.

PER SERVING: 98 calories, 3 g protein, 14 g carbohydrates, 2 g fiber, 4 g fat (0 g saturated), 6 mg sodium

STUFFED RICOTTA-AND-CHERRY PANCAKES

Prep time: 5 minutes / Total time: 1 hour 10 minutes /
Serve 8 (1 stuffed pancake per serving)

³/₄ cup white whole wheat flour or whole wheat pastry flour

2 egg whites

1 teaspoon canola oil

¹/₃ cup part-skim ricotta cheese

¹/₃ cup 0% fat plain Greek yogurt

3 teaspoons powdered sugar

1 teaspoon vanilla extract

1 cup fresh pitted cherries or frozen dark cherries, defrosted

1. Place the flour, egg whites, and oil in a blender. Blend until smooth and refrigerate for 1 hour.

2. Place the cheese, yogurt, 2 teaspoons of the sugar, and the vanilla extract in a medium bowl. Stir until well combined and then fold in the cherries. Refrigerate until ready to use.

3. Heat a large skillet or griddle over medium-high heat. Coat with cooking spray. Pour out about 3 tablespoons of the batter onto the griddle. Cook for 2 to 3 minutes, or until the edges of the pancake begin to crisp. Flip and cook 1 minute longer, or until the pancake is cooked through. Transfer to a plate and repeat with the remaining batter until you have 8 pancakes.

4. Divide the cheese mixture among the 8 pancakes and roll them up. Sprinkle with the remaining 1 teaspoon sugar and serve immediately.

PER SERVING: 101 calories, 5 g protein, 15 g carbohydrates, 0 g fiber, 2 g fat (1 g saturated), 45 mg sodium

SOFT CHOCOLATE CHIP COOKIES

Prep time: 5 minutes / Total time: 20 minutes /
Makes 2 dozen cookies (1 cookie per serving)

⅓ cup trans-free margarine, at room temperature

¾ cup light brown sugar, packed

1½ cups grated carrots (about 2 large carrots)

2 egg whites

2 tablespoons fat-free milk

1 teaspoon vanilla extract

½ cup bittersweet chocolate chips

1 cup white whole wheat flour or whole wheat pastry flour

¾ cup old-fashioned oats

1 teaspoon baking powder

1. Preheat the oven to 350°F. Coat 2 baking sheets with cooking spray. Place the margarine and brown sugar in a large bowl. Mash the brown sugar into the butter with a wooden spoon until combined.

2. Add the carrots, egg whites, milk, vanilla extract, and chocolate chips. Stir until combined.

3. Add the flour, oats, and baking powder to the mixture. Stir until a wet batter forms.

4. Drop the dough by tablespoonfuls onto the baking sheets and bake for 8 to 10 minutes, or until firm but not hard. Transfer the cookies to a wire rack to cool. Store in an airtight container for up to 4 days.

PER SERVING: 105 calories, 1 g protein, 15 g carbohydrates, 1 g fiber, 4 g fat (1 g saturated), 32 mg sodium

CHEF'S NOTE: Smart Balance is one good brand of trans-free margarine. Unlike most margarines, it doesn't have hydrogenated oil, and it bakes well. Avoid stone-ground whole wheat flour. White whole wheat and whole wheat pastry flour are more tender types of whole wheat flour. King Arthur and Arrowhead Mills, among other brands, make these types of flour.

PUMPKIN COOKIES WITH DRIED CHERRIES AND CREAM CHEESE ICING

Prep time: 5 minutes / Total time: 20 minutes / Makes 20 cookies (1 per serving)

1½	cups white whole wheat flour or whole wheat pastry flour
2	tablespoons ground flaxseed
1	teaspoon baking soda
1	teaspoon baking powder
¼	cup unsalted butter, at room temperature
½	cup light brown sugar, packed
½	cup pumpkin pie filling
1	egg
1	tablespoon molasses
½	cup dried cherries or cranberries
4	ounces low-fat cream cheese (½ block), at room temperature
1	tablespoon powdered sugar
2	tablespoons 0% fat plain Greek yogurt

1. Preheat the oven to 350°F. Coat 2 baking sheets with cooking spray.

2. Place the flour, flaxseed, baking soda, and baking powder in a large bowl. Whisk to combine.

3. Place the butter and sugar in another large bowl. Mash the sugar into the butter with a wooden spoon. Add the pie filling, egg, molasses, and cherries or cranberries and stir. Sprinkle the flour mixture over the top and stir until a thick batter forms.

4. Drop heaping teaspoons of the batter onto the baking sheets and bake for 8 to 10 minutes, or until the cookies are firm in the center. Transfer to a wire rack to cool completely.

5. Mash the cream cheese and powdered sugar together in a small bowl and stir in the yogurt. With a butter knife or small spatula, ice the cookies. Store in an airtight container for up to 3 days or freeze, tightly wrapped, for up to 3 months.

PER SERVING: 95 calories, 2 g protein, 14 g carbohydrates, 1 g fiber, 3 g fat (1 g saturated), 95 mg sodium

CHEF'S NOTE: Avoid stone-ground whole wheat flour. White whole wheat and whole wheat pastry flour are more tender types of whole wheat flour. King Arthur and Arrowhead Mills, among other brands, make these types of flour.

EASY ICE CREAM SANDWICHES

Prep time: 5 minutes / Total time: 2 hours /
Makes 8 ice cream sandwiches (1 per serving)

½ cup 0% fat plain Greek yogurt

½ pint fresh raspberries

¼ cup raspberry jam

3 tablespoons semisweet chocolate chips, chopped

8 thin store-bought chocolate wafers or thin cookies

1. Place the yogurt, raspberries, jam, and chocolate chips in a medium bowl. Stir until combined, mashing the raspberries with the back of the spoon.

2. Freeze, covered, for about 1 hour, or until the mixture begins to firm.

3. Line an airtight container with wax paper. Place half the wafers or cookies inside. With a small ice cream scoop, top each wafer with a scoop of the yogurt mixture. Top with another wafer and cover. Freeze for 1 hour longer, or until firm, and then serve.

PER SERVING: 109 calories, 2 g protein, 18 g carbohydrates, 1 g fiber, 3 g fat (1 g saturated), 5 mg sodium

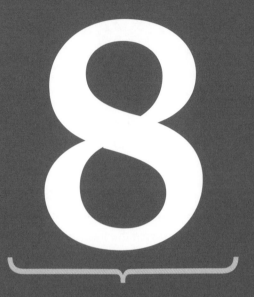

8

Get Out More:
Active Calories on the Go

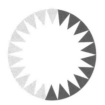

During the past 30 years, the number of calories the average American eats has risen from 1,826 a day to an
average of 2,157—an 18 percent, or 331-calorie, uptick.
Over the same 3-decade span, the average percentage of
daily meals eaten outside the home has seen nearly an
identical rise, from 18 percent to 37 percent. Coincidence? I think not.
Restaurant food is notoriously higher in sugar, salt, fat, and calories
than what we whip up on our own counters.

That's why preparing your own food is an essential part of Active
Calorie living. Whenever possible, I'd like you to be in your kitchen,
slicing and dicing and serving up home-cooked Active Calorie good-
ness. That said, if you're one of the women or men who currently eat
nearly 40 percent of their meals outside the home, you're not likely to
make a seismic shift overnight. I also understand that life can get pretty
hectic, and sometimes you're really in a rush, especially for breakfast
and lunch, which many of us eat on the run. That's why I've scoured
my resources to pinpoint the best Active Calorie options you'll find on
the road. I've included traditional fast food as well as a discussion of
"fast casual" food, like Così, Panera Bread, T.G.I. Friday's, and other sit-
down eateries. Plus, I've given you some pointers on what to eat at the

movies, the ballpark, and other hotspots where your food choices are limited.

The good news is that both fast and fast-casual foods have come a long way. Sure, you can still find diet bombs like triple cheeseburgers with extra bacon and 1,000-calorie taco salads. But you can also find truly healthy Active Calorie–worthy salads, sides, sandwiches, and entrées—even at the bar. Here's what to look for in popular nationwide chain restaurants (and, of course, you can apply these same principles when eating at your local deli, pub, and fine-dining establishments). Note that most restaurants also provide full nutritional info for their menu items online. Look them up on the Web, click the nutritional-info tab, and you'll find all the information you need to make smart, Active Calorie choices anywhere you go.

Fast Food

It's easy to go wrong—monumentally, Couch Potato Calorie wrong—with the 30-second, heat-lamp–warmed, drive-thru traditional fast-food fare like that stuffed into bags and handed through car windows at McDonald's and Taco Bell locations around the world. But thanks to demand from health-conscious customers like you, it's increasingly easier to get your food right.

This section will equip you to make smart Active Calorie choices on the go. That's not carte blanche to grab a sack of fast food every night of the week, however. I live in the real world and know that sometimes fast food is the only choice (or the preferred choice, even, in some situations). But limit yourself to no more than one or two fast-food meals a week. When you do stop for fast food, scan the menu for what you know are Active Calories: whole, recognizable foods; fresh vegetables and fruits; and lean meats like grilled chicken. Steer away from all those obvious Couch Potato Calories like french fries and processed foods like chicken patties on white buns. If you know that fast food is an inevitable part of your life, do as many of my clients do: Carry an apple or a banana, a small bag of baby carrots, or other portable fruits and/or vegetables with you. It'll save you money and give you an ever-ready healthy side no matter where you eat.

To give you an idea of what to look for when eating fast food, I scanned some of the menus of the most popular fast-food restaurants and picked good Active Calorie choices. Note that these do not follow the meal plan to the letter. In some cases, a meal may have more or fewer calories than generally recommended or occasionally may not have every element of the Active Calorie Diet represented. They're meant to be examples of meals that most closely embody the spirit of the Active Calorie Diet, with lean protein and fruits and vegetables for chewy and hearty calories. A number of these meals also have warming elements. I've provided examples for breakfast, lunch, dinner, and snacks/desserts where applicable (sometimes there really are no good choices). In general, lunch and dinner are interchangeable; just add a side or order a bit more food for dinner. Realize, of course, that restaurants (even fast-food chains) do change their menus. So use these as examples of the types of meals to order next time you have to grab and go.

Arby's

Arby's is obviously all about the roast beef, but honestly, none of the roast beef sandwiches are great Active Calorie choices. They have fair amounts of protein, but the food on this menu is pretty processed. Also beware the Market Fresh Sandwiches; they masquerade as Active Calorie options but are dietary land mines, with the healthy-looking Roast Turkey & Swiss packing 710 calories and the innocent-looking Ultimate BLT coming in at a walloping 820. Here are a few menu items to select.

LUNCH

Chopped Farmhouse Salad: Get it with roast chicken (not the spicy breaded option) and balsamic vinaigrette for a good Active Calorie meal at about 300 calories.

Roast Chicken Club Sandwich: Order without mayo and with extra Active Calorie toppings to bring this sandwich in at about 400 calories.

Burger King

The advice here is similar to that at McDonald's, though there may be less to choose from on the BK menu because it tends to cater to those who like their portions large.

LUNCH

BK Veggie Burger: As with the real deal, hold the mayo and order with extra lettuce and tomato.

Tendergrill Garden Salad: Ask them to hold the cheese on this salad and top with a light dressing instead.

Whopper Jr.: Despite the name, this isn't much of a whopper; it comes in at just over 300 calories. Order with no mayo and extra lettuce and tomato.

Chick-fil-A

Many of my clients believe that chicken is always inherently healthier than beef, which simply isn't true. There are a lot of ways to prepare poultry—breading and frying come to mind—that shift it into the Couch Potato Calorie direction. Fortunately, Chick-fil-A offers quite a few Active Calorie selections. As always, don't be shy about asking for extra lettuce, tomatoes, pickles, and Active Calorie toppings.

LUNCH

Chargrilled Chicken & Fruit Salad: This nice Active Calorie combo comes in under 300 calories and serves up a healthy portion of fruit in the form of apple slices, mandarin oranges, and strawberries, as well as veggies. There's some cheese, but they keep it light, so go ahead and sprinkle it around to enjoy the flavor. Order with the Berry Balsamic Vinaigrette for a warming Active Calorie bonus.

Chargrilled Chicken Sandwich: At 300 calories and with nearly 30 grams of protein, this sandwich is probably the best bet on the menu board. Add a side salad for a full meal.

SNACK OR DESSERT

Fruit Cup: Have a Fruit Cup on its own as a snack, or add one to any meal to make up an Active Calorie Plate. But beware the Carrot & Raisin Salad. It looks innocent and healthy but is loaded with sugar and actually adds nearly 400 calories to your meal.

KFC

The Colonel's secret recipe can be one for waistline (and cardiac-health) disaster. Fried, deep-fried, and extra-crispy food is all over the menu. But KFC is trying to promote its "unfried side." So look a little closer and you'll find there are a few selections on the lighter, Active Calorie side.

LUNCH

Honey BBQ Sandwich: This Southern specialty is just over 300 calories. Get it with a side of green beans and corn on the cob (not smothered in butter).

Toasted Wrap with Tender Roast Filet: You can get this sandwich for less than 300 calories if you hold the sauce. Then add corn and green beans as sides.

DINNER

Grilled Chicken BLT Salad: Go easy on the bacon, heavy on the tomato, and order with light Italian dressing for a filling dinner salad.

McDonald's

The key to eating well at the Golden Arches is choosing items that are of reasonable portions and seeking out the word *grilled* on the menu. And say "no, thanks" when asked if you want fries with your order. The chain has made a concerted effort to add some healthful items. By choosing them, you'll encourage more of the same.

BREAKFAST

Egg McMuffin: Order it with Canadian-style bacon instead of sausage. Have an orange juice or, better yet, apple slices on the side.

LUNCH

Plain hamburger: This is the small patty, folks. Ask for extra lettuce and tomato.

Southwest Salad with Grilled Chicken: Go easy on the dressing and have with a side of apple slices.

Premium Grilled Chicken Classic: Be sure to specify no mayo. Ask for extra lettuce and tomato.

SNACK AND DESSERT

Fruit 'N Yogurt Parfait: I would make this heavier on the fruit and lighter on the granola, but it's not bad as is. It's made with low-fat yogurt.

Snack Size Fruit and Walnut Salad: At about 200 calories, this could be a nice addition (way better than fries) to a plain burger for a larger meal.

Pizza Hut

Notorious for turning dietary bombs into nuclear disasters (meat lover's pie with cheese-stuffed crust, anyone?), Pizza Hut's menu is loaded to the gills with thousands of Couch Potato Calories. But all hope is not lost the moment you walk under that bright red roof. Scan the menu board and you'll find a few Active Calorie items that will let you join the party without wrecking your waist.

LUNCH

Thin 'N Crispy Veggie Lover's Pizza (1 slice): Not quite as lean as the chain's Fit 'n Delicious line but not too bad, either. The Veggie Lover's (and Ham and Pineapple) variety comes in at 240 calories a slice. Add a salad with light vinaigrette for a complete meal.

DINNER

12" Fit 'n Delicious Pizza (2 slices): Most Pizza Huts offer a line of health-conscious pies that have half the cheese, more veggies, and lean meats and come in at 150 to 180 calories per slice. The options: Chicken, Red Onion & Green Pepper; Chicken, Mushrooms & Jalapeño; Ham, Red Onion & Mushroom; Ham, Pineapple & Diced Red Tomato; Green Pepper, Red Onion & Diced Red Tomato; and Diced Red Tomato, Mushroom & Jalapeño. Any of them fit into your plan. You can add a salad with light vinaigrette to those that are a little lower in calories. Choose the ones with a little heat via the peppers for extra Active Calorie points.

Quiznos

Quiznos prides itself on having a vast under-500 menu, so that's a great starting point. Obviously, not everything in that selection is necessarily good for you. But you can find some reasonable selections for sure. Here are a few to try.

LUNCH

Cantina Chicken Flatbread: Bring a Greek yogurt and an apple to round out your meal.

Chili: This meaty, beany chili is packed with protein and fiber, making it a great Active Calorie choice.

Pesto Turkey Toasty Bullet: This little sandwich—with tangy red wine vinaigrette and plenty of lettuce, tomato, and basil pesto—is an Active Calorie winner.

Raspberry Vinaigrette Chicken: Grilled chicken on a bed of lettuce and other veggies makes for a balanced Active Calorie meal.

Subway

Thanks to longtime Subway spokesman Jared, this sandwich chain became synonymous with weight loss through fast food. There are many healthful choices on the menu, but don't make the mistake of thinking that just because it's from Subway, it's all Active Calorie approved. A macadamia nut cookie is still 220 Couch Potato Calories that you don't need; though the chips are generally baked, they're still potato chips; and a soda is a soda, no matter what shop sells it. Here are some of the best items on the menu.

LUNCH

Fresh Fit 6″ Subs: It's hard to go wrong with Subway's Fresh Fit menu, which features eight sandwiches—including Ham,

Oven Roasted Chicken, Sweet Onion Chicken Teriyaki, Turkey Breast, and Veggie Delite—that have fewer than 6 grams of fat and come in under 400 calories. You'll notice that these sandwiches don't have cheese (a quick calorie booster), so don't add any if you want to keep the calorie count low. Load up on lettuce and tomatoes. To add heat, feel free to pile on the peppers or add a splash of vinegar and a sprinkle of pepper.

SNACK OR DESSERT

Mini Subs: Another smart Active Calorie option is to order one of Subway's Mini Subs (it offers ham, roast beef, turkey, and veggie, all of which are just 200 calories or less). Remember that cheese and creamy dressings quickly add unwanted calories. Go light on the cheese, and choose vinaigrettes and Active Calorie toppings like veggies. If you want to have one for lunch, pair it with one of the healthier soups. The Rosemary Chicken and Dumpling has just 90 calories, as do the Minestrone and Tomato Garden Vegetable with Rotini.

Taco Bell

"Taco Bell" and "Active Calorie eating" were not two phrases you'd use in the same sentence a few years back. To the chain's credit, it has crossed the border into far healthier food with the Fresco line. When you order something "fresco," they replace the cheese and fatty sauce with fresh salsa and cilantro, which fill nearly all your Active Calorie needs. You can pair any of these with beans for more filling fiber.

LUNCH OR DINNER

Fresco Burrito Supreme: Order any of the Supreme Burritos fresco and add extra salsa and lettuce. Whether you go with chicken or steak, your meal still comes in at around 330 calories.

Fresco Crunchy Taco: At just 150 calories, you can get your Mexican fast-food fix while doing nearly nil dietary damage. Have two with added beans for lunch or dinner.

Fresco Grilled Steak Soft Taco: Slightly more calories but about half the fat of a crunchy taco. This is a pretty good Active Calorie choice. Have two with added beans for lunch or dinner.

Fresco Ranchero Chicken Soft Taco: Even fewer fat calories than the Grilled Steak Soft Taco. Have two with added beans for lunch or dinner.

Fresco Tostada: A flat corn shell topped with fiber-rich beans makes this a healthy Active Calorie alternative to the usual cheesy, fatty fare. Have two with added beans for lunch or dinner.

Grilled Chicken Taquitos: A little higher in fat than I'd like, but if you need a change, not a bad choice at 320 calories overall.

Wendy's

Their burgers tend to tilt heavy on the calorie scale, but there are quite a few other meals to choose from that will help you stay on the Active Calorie track.

LUNCH

Apple Pecan Chicken Salad: Made with grilled chicken, this is a good chewy and hearty choice. Just go easy on the dressing.

Baja Salad: Order without the cheese, and you have a complete, filling meal, along with a dash of warming Active Calories.

Grilled Chicken Go Wrap: It's hard to recommend many of Wendy's burgers, since even the small one is pretty high on

BUZZ WORDS AND BAD WORDS

THE MENU SUGGESTIONS in this chapter will get you pointed in the right direction. But let's face it: Eventually you're going to find yourself in your local mom-and-pop diner or other eatery that didn't make this list. You need to know how to scan a menu for words that indicate whether what you're ordering is an Active Calorie food or laden with Couch Potato Calories. Here's what to look for from each list.

ACTIVE CALORIE DESCRIPTIONS*

Baked	Light	Reduced	Vinaigrette
Boiled	Marinated	Roasted	Whole wheat
Broiled	Poached	Steamed	
Grilled	Red sauce	Stir-fried	

*Even if you see these words on the menu, you still have to check for butter and creamy sauces, which can tip these dishes into Couch Potato territory.

COUCH POTATO CALORIE DESCRIPTIONS

Au gratin	Buttery	Creamy	Smothered
Basted	Casserole	Crispy	Stroganoff
Battered	Cheesy	Fried	White sauce
Breaded	Country-style	Loaded	

the calorie scale. At under 300 calories and stuffed with some veggies, this wrap is a smart Active Calorie choice.

Jr. Hamburger: This is the only burger that falls within a reasonable 300-calorie range. Get it with extra lettuce and tomato and no mayo.

Small Chili and Baked Potato: Order without cheese or sour cream, and eat the potato skin for extra fiber. Eat just half the potato; save the other half for later. Add mandarin oranges for extra fruit.

Ultimate Chicken Grill: Another good choice from Wendy's. This sandwich comes with honey mustard sauce instead of mayo. As always, ask for extra lettuce and tomato.

Fast Casual

Fast-casual eateries like T.G.I. Friday's, Così, and Panera Bread have been the fastest-growing segment of the restaurant industry for years. A recent report shows that 25 percent of their customers are women who work outside the home and 15 percent are stay-at home moms. I understand the appeal of these establishments. Fast casuals are generally a step up from fast food in both food quality and eating atmosphere. The food comes relatively fast and is modestly priced, and children are welcome.

But you can get in trouble quickly because many of the dishes that look Active Calorie friendly are Couch Potato Calories in disguise. It's also very, very easy to eat hundreds, if not thousands (yes, thousands), more calories than you intend at these places, since some dishes that look light are actually caloric heavyweights, coming in at 1,000 or more per entrée. What's more, I've found that in too many cases, the healthy options they do offer are bland and tasteless. A co-worker recently ordered a side of grilled asparagus at a Ruby Tuesday that was shriveled, stiff, and all but inedible. It was so bad, she couldn't even finish 10 stalks, and she loves asparagus.

As with any time you eat out, you need to be cautious. The good news is that many of these establishments are making sincere attempts to offer fresher, healthier, lower-calorie fare that tastes good, too. Here, I have tried to provide a snapshot of the type of items you'll find in some of the most popular fast-casual eateries and advice on how to choose wisely. Because the menus often vary by region and change frequently, I provided only a handful of specific Active Calorie dishes. Instead, my intent is to give you the tools you need to walk in and confidently choose a meal that fits your Active Calorie life—a meal that contains whole foods and an array of CHEW Active Calories. As with fast food, try to limit the number of meals eaten at fast-casual eateries to no more than one, maybe two, per week. Here's the lowdown on what to look for (also check out "Buzz Words and Bad Words" on page 203 to assist you in making choices).

Applebee's

The self-proclaimed king of the fast-casual genre, it has more than 2,000 restaurants in 49 states. Applebee's has done an admirable job creating a flavorful menu that meets many of the Active Calorie standards. In fact, the Spicy Shrimp Diavolo, part of the Under 550 Calories menu, has protein, vegetables, whole grain carbs, and, of course, warming spices. Check out the other healthful Under 550 Calories choices, including Grilled Shrimp & Island Rice, Asian Crunch Salad, Grilled Dijon Chicken & Portobellos, and Asiago Peppercorn Steak. Applebee's has also joined forces with Weight Watchers to create a few signature dishes that won't crack your WW "points" budget. It's best to avoid dishes not on the WW or Under 550 list, because their calorie count is apt to be sky high—especially of the Couch Potato variety.

Chili's

My first advice for anyone eating at Chili's is to skip all the appetizers. Many of them push past the 1,000-calorie range—Texas Cheese Fries with Chili and Jalapeño Ranch dressing, for example, enter the whopping 2,000-calorie range! Instead, start with the Guiltless Grill menu. But be warned, the chain defines "guiltless" as having fewer than 750 calories, which doesn't always match my definition, especially when many of those calories are the Couch Potato kind. The good news is, these items are all made to order, so you can activate any dish by adding veggies and removing excess starch or fat. Chili's also has a

(continued on page 208)

{ deborah griffin }

His Couch Potato Calories
Made Her Put on Pounds

AGE: 40
POUNDS LOST:
9.4
INCHES LOST:
4 1/2 including 2 3/4 off her waist

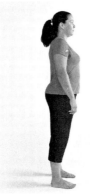

BEFORE

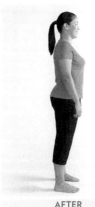

AFTER

IT'S WELL DOCUMENTED that men and women tend to put on weight once they're in a committed relationship. There are lots of reasons for that. They tend to eat out more often. Life gets busy. They have kids. They're not dating, so they let their food guards down a little. Deborah "Debe" Griffin was a little different. "My boyfriend runs marathons," she bemoaned. "We're eating together now. He can eat a box of pasta and burn it off. I'm not burning it off. But I just can't seem to stick to one serving size, either." The result: She had gained 30 pounds in the past year.

Obviously I didn't want Debe to break up with her boyfriend! But she needed a solution. Debe's boyfriend ate carbs—a lot of carbs, all the time. She was doing the same. She needed something more filling so she wouldn't be tempted to polish off his gargantuan portions of pasta, but also something that wouldn't fill her out. Active Calories to the rescue: She added protein to her breakfast. "I'd never eaten protein in the morning," she recalls. Likewise, she put more veggies and protein on her dinner plate so there'd be less room for starch. The rewards were nearly instantaneous. In 1 week I got the happy news: "I started last Tuesday, and I wanted to let you know that I lost 3 pounds almost immediately, so I am very excited! Thank you!"

It just kept getting better from there. Debe decided to turn this plan into a personal challenge to make sustainable changes for long-term weight loss. "I've lost about 10 pounds so far, and it's a very satisfying diet. Every night I look into my fridge to see how many vegetables I can stuff into whatever I'm making. It's fun—a good challenge." She also started experimenting with sweeteners, such as agave, to add to her yogurt for a more active dessert than ice cream. She also loves how the Active Calorie Diet is expanding her tastes.

"All I can say is, wow, just wow," she raved during her final weigh-in. "My stomach actually felt concave yesterday morning.

"This is a diet I can definitely live with. I'll be honest—the first day was a little overwhelming because I was trying to figure out what to buy and prepare and eat. But after that, it became automatic. I love how active it makes me feel. Plus, the results are so worth it! I also love that I now know how to eat no matter where I am. We went to Golden Corral, and I knew even there how to put together a good, healthy plate of food. This is something my whole family can do. It's great."

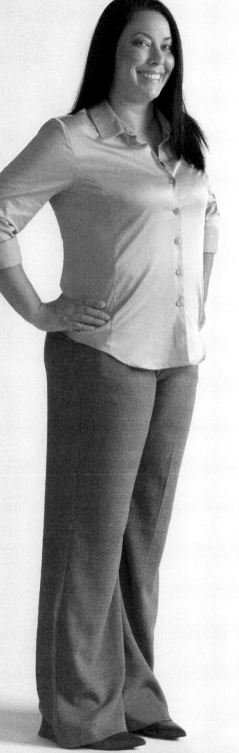

complete vegetarian menu that you can download from the Web site. (You can swap a black bean burger for a beef patty in the burger selections.) Other smart choices include the Guiltless Grilled Salmon, the Guiltless Chicken Platter, and the Guiltless Grill Pita.

Così

This is a favorite family joint among my co-workers. The soups, with the exception of the New England Clam Chowder, are all within a reasonable calorie range and come with whole grain flatbread. The salads are creative (just watch the sometimes heavy dressings)—I especially like the Shanghai Chicken; its ginger dressing also adds some warming Active Calories. The Fire-Roasted Veggie sandwich is brimming with vegetables, coated with a savory feta cheese spread, and still has only 324 calories. Check out the Our Lighter Side menu for dishes designed to be easier on your waistline. Sides include baby carrots and fresh fruit. You can even wash it all down with freshly brewed green teas for some energizing Active Calories.

Noodles & Company

With a name that has "Noodles" right up front and center, you'd think this would be so starch-centric that it would be strictly off-limits for the Active Calorie plan. But this creative chain works very hard to accommodate every smart eater's concerns. Right on its Web site, you can find dishes for people watching fat, calories, sodium, or carbs or who have allergies. Every dish is made to order, so you can freely swap or add veggies and protein and turn up the heat with a variety of spices—ideal for the Active Calorie plan. You can pair Pad Thai with a small Chinese Chop Salad for a really tasty 500-calorie meal. Or go with one of the Trios, such as Japanese Pan Noodles with Shrimp and Tossed Green Side Salad with Fat-Free Asian Dressing for 415 calories or Bangkok Curry with Shrimp and Tossed Green Side Salad with Fat-Free Asian Dressing for just 310 calories.

Olive Garden

I'm sure I don't need to tell you that there's really not much room for bottomless pasta bowls and a steady stream of breadsticks (they're 140 calories apiece and go down as quickly as they're replenished, so you can actually lose count) in the Active Calorie Diet. But that doesn't mean that Olive Garden is off-limits. Far from it, actually. Just stick with the Garden Fare, a special menu that is designed to serve specific dietary needs, particularly low fat and low carb (and generally low calorie). Some good Active Calorie choices include Venetian Apricot Chicken, which is topped with an apricot citrus sauce and comes with sides of broccoli, asparagus, and diced tomatoes; Grilled Chicken Spiedini, which is marinated in Italian herbs and olive oil and served with grilled veggies and Tuscan potatoes; Herb-Grilled Salmon with broccoli; and the classic Minestrone soup, which is brimming with filling Active Calories in the form of fresh vegetables and beans. If it's not on the Garden Fare menu, I'd simply avoid it entirely. So many of the dishes have more than 1,000 calories and are loaded with creamy, buttery, cheesy sauces.

Outback Steakhouse

With its famous 1,500-calorie Bloomin' Onion and a Queensland Salad that sets you back an astonishing 1,074 calories, Outback is no bastion of healthy eating. It offers no special lighter-fare menu options. But this Aussie-themed eatery is not without merit. Its no-rules policy allows customers to request meals made to their liking, so you can easily switch out a starchy side for steamed veggies. The steaks were rated number one best steak in the 2009 Zagat Survey of National Full-Service Restaurant Chains, and you can enjoy a 6-ounce Outback Special for just 330 calories. Add steamed, seasoned green beans without the butter for another 50 calories, and you have a pretty decent Active Calorie Plate. As a matter of fact, they like their butter a lot at Outback, so you can shave at least 100 calories off many menu items simply by saying, "No butter, please."

MEAL REPLACEMENTS

THERE ARE TIMES WHEN YOU may be tied to your desk and tempted to reach for a meal-replacement bar or shake to chow down and plow ahead. Don't do it. These processed, packaged foods do not count as Active Calories. Yes, some of them have fiber and protein and are infused with vitamins and minerals. But my experience is that these products don't provide enough substance to be satisfying, so people eat or drink them, then eat twice as much later on. Sure, if the choice is a Snickers or a Balance Bar, the Balance Bar is a better choice—but one to be made only in an extreme pinch, not as a habit.

Panera Bread

I applaud Panera for using antibiotic-free chicken and fresh ingredients in its dishes. I also love the creative, seasonal salads that feature a medley of fruits, veggies, and tangy dressings. Just remember that even if it's artisanal, Three Cheese bread is still loaded with Couch Potato Calories, as are many of the thick, rich, buttery soups and sides. Look for dishes that are clearly labeled "low fat" or are obviously chock-full of Active Calorie ingredients. I like the Mediterranean Veggie on Tomato Basil sandwich and Low-Fat Vegetarian Black Bean soup. Many of the sandwiches come smeared with a heavy brush of mayo, so be sure to ask for mustard instead.

P. F. Chang's

As at any Chinese restaurant, you'll find your share of greasy fat bombs. But you'll also find some delicious lighter fare. This Asian chain serves up a full gluten-free menu and vegetarian items, and you can ask for dishes made to order. Like most fast-casual eateries, this one allows you to check the calorie counts of all its dishes online. My one beef: They're printed according to serving size instead of simply according to the entire dish (which is really what you're ordering, right?). I suggest getting creative and making a full Active Calorie meal out of appetizers and sides.

For instance, the Seared Ahi Tuna (220 calories), Hot and Sour Soup (56 calories), and Garlic Snap Peas (120 calories) make for a delicious, savory meal with plenty of heat that comes in at around just 400 calories.

Red Lobster

Many of my clients make the mistake of thinking that just because it's fish or seafood, it's gotta be good for you. That's mostly true, until you take that sea creature and drop it in butter, breading, and a deep fryer! At Red Lobster, that describes a hearty chunk of the menu. In fact, you can get entire dishes that are nothing but various shapes of golden brown breading. Fortunately, the chain also offers lighter fare in the form of the LightHouse Menu. What's on the menu varies from region to region, but typical dishes include Live Maine Lobster with a potato topped with pico de gallo (far better than butter and includes warming Active Calories!) and a Garden Salad with balsamic vinaigrette, all for just 430 calories; a variety of wood-grilled fresh fish, including salmon, trout, and tilapia; and Chilled Jumbo Shrimp Cocktail. Avoid the salads, which tend to be loaded up with cheese, fatty dressing, croutons, and other fried things, and go with the fresh vegetable sides, like broccoli and asparagus, instead.

Ruby Tuesday

Like many fast-casual chains, Ruby Tuesday recognizes that there are people who want lower-calorie, health-friendly choices when they eat out. That's nice, especially from a chain whose handcrafted and premium burgers all crack the 1,000-calorie range. In that vein, it has created a Fit & Trim menu. Problem is, the chain's definition of "fit and trim" is meals that come in under 700 calories, a few of which—like the Herb Crusted Tilapia, which comes with white Cheddar mashed potatoes and steamed broccoli—wouldn't exactly top my list of Active Calorie choices. Many of the Fit & Trim meals, like the otherwise decent Petite Sirloin (561 calories), also come with bland or, worse, sort of bitter vegetable sides like steamed broccoli that wouldn't inspire anyone to ask for more. So choose wisely. Your best bet may be the salad bar, which generally offers ample healthy fruit and vegetable options.

T.G.I. Friday's

Much of T.G.I. Friday's menu is a true Active Calorie Diet disaster. Even the salads come in at 700 calories, with all the cheese and dressing and fried things in and on them. So you need to approach this chain's menu with a very careful eye. Ironically, the items on the Jack Daniel's Grill signature menu may be your best bet because they're grilled. Barbecue Jack Chicken and Jack Daniel's Chicken and Shrimp can be turned into decent Active Calorie Plates if you order them without butter and with veggies rather than mashed potatoes. Other relatively safe choices include the Shrimp Key West and the Santa Fe Chopped Salad with chicken (get the dressing on the side). Skip most of the appetizers because they're fried and fat-filled.

Out and About

Where there's life, there's food, usually in abundance and often not terribly good for you. But whether you're out at the movies or spending the afternoon at the ballgame, you don't need to succumb to the call of Couch Potato Calories. Look closely and you can generally (but I'll be honest, not always) find an Active Calorie alternative that will satisfy your need to snack while keeping your weight loss goals on track. I also recommend having a healthy meal before you go, so you're less susceptible to mindless munching and poor food choices.

The following are some smart Active Calorie selections to go with the entertainment of your choice.

At the Movies

This could be the place with the paltriest Active Calorie choices. Sure, popcorn is chewy and fairly rich in fiber. But movie theater popcorn packs a stunning number of calories—more than 650 for the smallest serving! Why? Because it's oil, not air, popped. Add butter and you dump on another 200 Couch Potato Calories. If you need to munch with your matinee, I highly recommend bringing a small snack pack of baby carrots or even a zip-top bag of your own air-popped popcorn. Otherwise, stick to the smallest treat you can find and split it with friends.

At the Ballpark

Sports stadiums have come a long way from the days when they served up nothing but hotdogs and beer. Today's ballpark concessions offer sushi, paninis, and plenty of Active Calorie fare. Take a lap around; bypass the nachos, cheese fries, and other Couch Potato fare and go for a chicken sandwich, sushi, or even a plain burger instead.

At the Fair

We've all heard about the fried Twinkies and other lard-bombs offered at fair food vendors around the country. Amid the deep-fried fodder, however, you can find plenty of healthy food at a fair, including corn on the cob, gyros, and grilled chicken. If you live for funnel cake, don't deprive yourself of a once-a-year treat. Buy one and split it among your family and friends so you all have a taste but no one overdoes it.

At the Bar

The same rules apply at the bar that apply in fast casual eateries (see page 204). Skip the mozzarella sticks, wings, jalapeño poppers, and other fried, fatty fare. Opt instead for shrimp cocktail, a pita and hummus, chicken satay, even soft tacos (light on the cheese, no sour cream). These are all acceptable Active Calorie choices. Want a beer or cocktail? Go ahead and have one. Just avoid drinks made with high-calorie mixers, and make sure your next beverage is water, unsweetened green tea, or another Active Calorie drink.

9

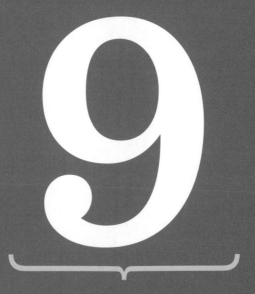

Move More:
The Active Calorie Workout

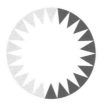

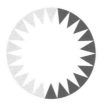A ctivity. It's the bread and butter (or, rather, baguette and olive oil) of the Active Calorie Diet. Active Calories aren't just active in the way your body digests and uses them; they are also the perfect fuel for a vibrant, active life. This type of eating makes you a better fat-burner (as described earlier, your body gradually adjusts to burn the fuel you feed it most often), which means that the activity you do will burn more fat.

Though the Active Calorie plan isn't an exercise program, I recommend including daily activity to speed your results and improve your health. Research proves that if you want to be trim, eating less will place you on the right path, but adding exercise puts you in the fast lane. Getting your rear in gear will also make it easier to resist those Couch Potato Calories. Exercise triggers dopamine, a chemical that governs your brain's reward center, as well as those feel-good brain chemicals called endorphins, so you're less likely to find your hands rustling at the bottom of a bag of chips—or Dove chocolates—to lift your mood. Just 10 minutes of exercise a day is enough to trip your brain's pleasure center and ward off unhealthy cravings, according to research from the University of Exeter in Britain.[1] Regular exercise can also help you eat less by suppressing your appetite. A review article by

Tufts University researchers concluded that people who exercise enjoy a "spontaneous reduction in hunger."[2]

Most important, combining healthy eating with regular physical activity not only feels good but also is good for you. In a recent study from Louisiana State University, researchers had one group of over-weight volunteers cut calories by 25 percent, while the other group used a combination of diet and exercise to reduce their daily calories by the same amount. At the end of 6 months, both groups had lost about 10 percent of their body weight, but only the exercisers enjoyed improvements in their blood pressure, insulin sensitivity, and choles-terol levels.[3]

Keeping It Off

Though you can lose weight through diet alone, if you want to keep those pounds gone for good, exercise is essential. The National Weight Control Registry reports that 90 percent of dieters who succeed in keeping off the lost weight exercise almost daily.

More interesting, exercise appears to be especially potent at keep-ing dangerous belly fat at bay. In one study, researchers put 97 women on a very low-calorie diet until the women had lost about 27 pounds. The researchers then put some of the women on a walking program and others on a strength-training plan and told the rest to do no exer-cise at all. All of the women resumed their old eating habits. The women who continued exercising regained less weight than those who didn't, which is no surprise. What was surprising was that the exercis-ers didn't regain weight around their waistlines, while the nonexercis-ers not only regained their weight but also packed it on, mostly around their middles.[4]

Scientists are still sorting out the whys of this weight-regaining phenomenon, but animal studies suggest that it's because exercise trains your body to metabolize calories differently. In lab experiments in which mice ran on wheels to shed pounds, they became better fat-burners (which we know is also true for exercising humans). They also tended to burn fat immediately after their meals, while their slothful counterparts burned carbs and were more likely to send fat off to be stored in fat cells. Exercising animals also appeared to be satisfied with less food. All of those adaptations have made scientists speculate that regular exercise might help reestablish your "set point," the weight that your body decides to defend. In short, exercise may help you burn more fat, eat less, and stay slimmer once the weight is gone. Sounds good to me.

Move Every Muscle: Active Calorie Strength Training

The focus of the plan is the Active Calorie resistance-training workout— a six-move strength-training routine that targets multiple body parts, like your arms and legs, simultaneously. This multimuscle technique builds strength, tones muscle, and burns more calories overall in less workout time. Each of these moves also has a balance challenge, so while you're working your arms, legs, butt, chest, and back, your core will be constantly engaged, giving you a special core-strengthening bonus. More important, because these moves mimic the way you use your body every day, they train your muscles to work in unison the way you use them in the real world and give you what we call functional fitness: the strength and stamina you need to juggle a squirming 25-pound toddler in one arm and a 10-pound grocery bag in the other, while somehow fishing keys from your pocket and dashing to the door because said toddler "really has to go."

Do the strength moves 2 or 3 days a week (but not on back-to-back days; your muscles need a day off in between to recover and repair). Do two sets of 8 to 12 reps of each exercise before moving to the next. You'll feel the difference immediately, and you'll see results in 2 to

ONE-TWO PUNCH FOR COUCH POTATO CALORIES

STRENGTH TRAINING IS A PERFECT ANTIDOTE to Couch Potato Calories. In one study, Syracuse University researchers found that a single weight-training session reduced the blood-sugar spiking effect of a high-sugar meal by 15 percent for more than 12 hours afterward.[5] The likely reason: Strength training drains your muscles' fuel reserves (known as glycogen stores). To ensure that your muscles have the energy they need for whatever you do next, your body immediately pulls any available glucose out of your bloodstream and into your muscles, where it's packed away for future use. Because vigorous aerobic exercise taps your glycogen stores, too, you can get a similar benefit from energetic cardio sessions.

4 weeks. If you're picking up dumbbells for the first time, here are some strength-training basics. The word *rep* is short for repetition: For example, each time you lift and lower a dumbbell or roll your upper body off the floor and then lower it back down, it's considered 1 repetition. A specific number of reps (8, 10, 12, and so on) is called a set.

If you have never done any strength-training exercises (or haven't exercised in more than 6 months) or you're simply having trouble maintaining good form, start with the "Make It Easier" option. If you're experienced at strength training or a move is not challenging enough, perform the "Make It Harder" option.

For the best results, the weight you choose should be heavy enough that by your last rep, you feel as if you can't do any more using good form. If you can't do at least 8 reps, then the weight is too heavy. Choose a lighter weight. Because some muscles are bigger than others, you'll need to use heavier weights for exercises that target your chest, back, legs, and butt. For smaller muscles, like your arms and shoulders, you'll probably want lighter weights. If you are a beginner, start with 3- and 5-pound dumbbells. Advanced exercisers can start with 5- to 8-pound dumbbells.

{ kim wagner }

Meds No More!

AGE: 33

POUNDS LOST:
8.2

INCHES LOST:
6¼ including 3½ off her thighs

WHEN TEST PANELIST Kim Wagner first came to see me, she didn't know how to cook or shop. She and her boyfriend just ate out—and not well. Around the house, they ate junk food and candy. The toll on her health wasn't pretty—too many unwanted pounds and daily medication for diabetes.

Kim was nervous to start but very happy to report that learning how to shop and eat the Active Calorie way was not as hard as she had feared. She and her boyfriend now cook in more often than they eat out, and they've enjoyed trying new foods so much that she went onto YouTube to find new cooking ideas.

"Information is powerful," she told me during our final check-in. By knowing what to put on her plate (and what not to), she didn't have to worry about counting calories. And she still lost weight. Best of all, she no longer needs her diabetes medications. She has been running and was set to tackle her first 10-K shortly after the check-in. And she's going to keep going. She and her boyfriend are set to continue following the plan, and Kim is signing up for a half-marathon in May. Now, that's an Active Calorie transformation!

step and extend

TONES: Glutes, legs, arms, and shoulders

1. Holding the dumbbells at your shoulders, palms facing in, stand facing a staircase. Plant your right foot on the first step. (You can use the second or third step, depending on the height of the stairs and your fitness level.)

2. Press into your right foot and straighten the right leg while lifting the weights overhead. Tap your left toes on the step, then lower both feet back to the starting position. Complete a full set. Switch legs for your second set.

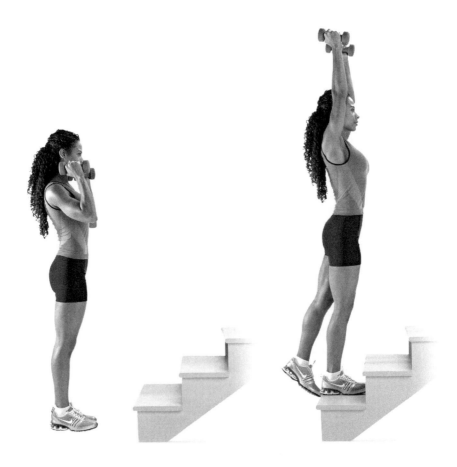

MAKE IT EASIER: Perform the move without the overhead press.

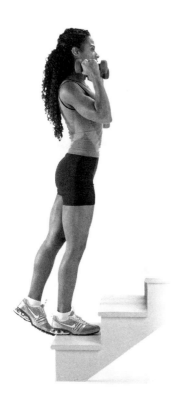

MAKE IT HARDER: Keep the foot you're stepping up with planted on the step throughout the exercise (lowering just the other foot to the floor).

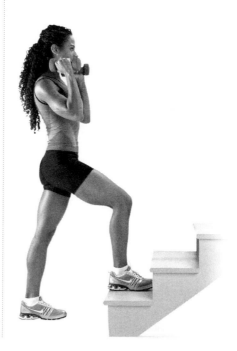

split squat, biceps curl

TONES: Glutes, legs, arms, and core

1. Stand with your right leg 2 to 3 feet in front of your left leg. Hold a pair of dumbbells down at your sides.

2. Bend your right leg until your right thigh is parallel to the floor and the left leg is extended, with the knee slightly bent and almost touching the floor. Be sure to keep your back straight, and don't allow your right knee to jut beyond your right toes. As you lower, bend your arms and curl the weights to your chest. Pause, then push back up to the starting position, lowering the weights as you stand. Complete a full set. Switch leg positions for your second set.

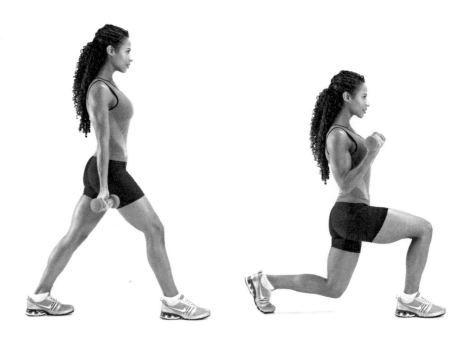

MAKE IT EASIER: Place one hand on a chair back for balance, and curl with only one arm at a time.

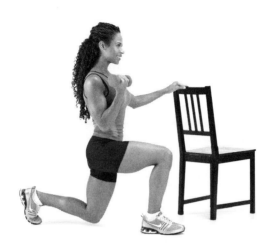

MAKE IT HARDER: Place the top of your back foot on a step.

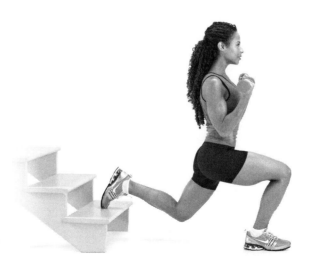

single-leg row

TONES: Glutes, legs, back, arms, and shoulders

1. Stand with your feet hip-width apart, holding the dumbbells down at your sides, palms facing in.

2. Bend forward toward the floor while extending your left leg straight behind you until your body forms a T (or as close to it as possible). Allow your arms to hang straight down toward the floor, with your palms facing each other.

3. Squeeze your shoulder blades together and raise the weights to either side of your chest. Repeat for half a set, then switch sides.

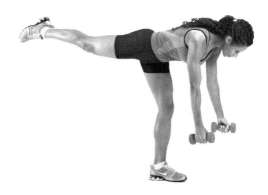

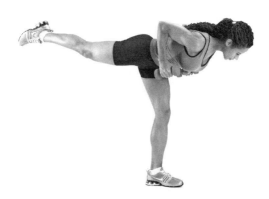

MAKE IT EASIER: Hold on to a chair back with one hand, and perform the rows one arm at a time.

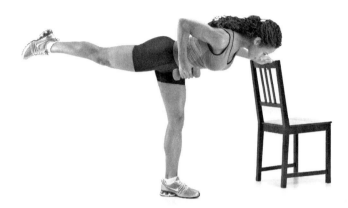

MAKE IT HARDER: After rowing the weights to your chest, extend your arms straight back to add a triceps kick-back.

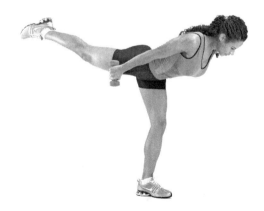

flamingo lateral lift

TONES: Shoulders, glutes, and core

1. Stand with your feet hip-width apart. Hold the dumbbells down at your sides, with your palms facing in.

2. Bend your right leg and lift your right foot off the floor as high as comfortably possible while maintaining your balance. Tighten your glutes and abs for support, and slowly lift the weights straight out to the sides until your arms are parallel to the floor. Lower your arms back to the starting position, and repeat for a full set. Switch legs for the second set.

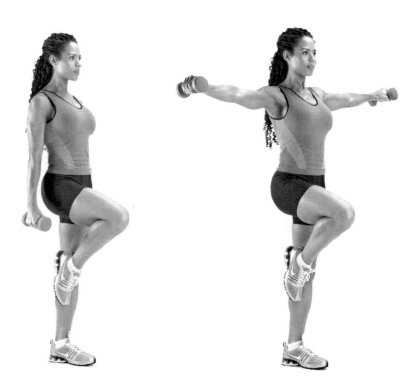

MAKE IT EASIER: Lightly place one foot on a step instead of suspending it in the air.

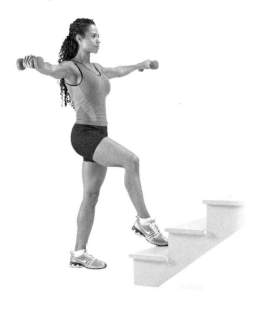

MAKE IT HARDER: Extend the lifted leg, holding it as high as possible while maintaining good form.

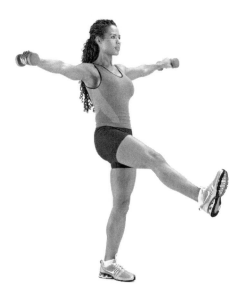

dip and crunch

TONES: Arms, shoulders, and abs

1. Sit on the edge of a chair with your feet flat on the floor and your knees bent 90 degrees. Grasp the chair seat on either side of your butt. Walk your feet out slightly and inch yourself off the seat. Extend your right leg and plant the heel on the ground, keeping your foot flexed.

2. Bend your elbows straight back and dip your butt toward the ground while simultaneously contracting your abs and pulling your right knee toward your chest. Don't dip your elbows past 90 degrees. Return to the starting position. Complete a set (you may not be able to do 10 the first few times). Switch legs for the second set.

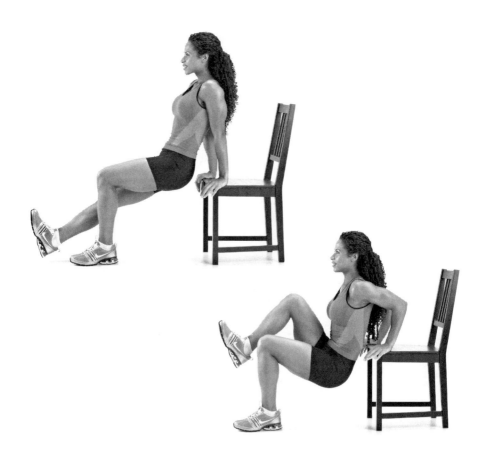

THE ACTIVE CALORIE DIET

MAKE IT EASIER: Keep both legs bent while performing the move.

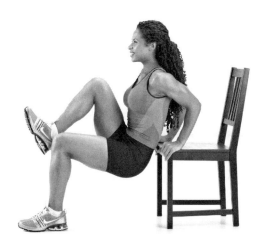

MAKE IT HARDER: Extend both legs while performing the move, bending the leg you bring to your chest.

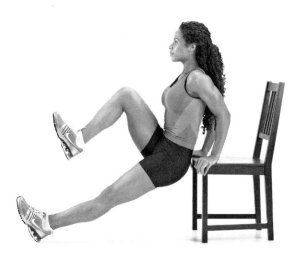

chest-press punch

TONES: Core, chest, shoulders, and arms

1. Lie on your back on a mat or carpeted floor and bend your knees. Hold two dumbbells at either side of your chest, with the ends facing each other.

2. Contract your abs and curl your head, shoulders, and torso off the floor. As you come up, extend your right arm across your body to the left as though throwing a light punch in that direction. Return to the starting position. Repeat on the opposite side. Alternate for a full set.

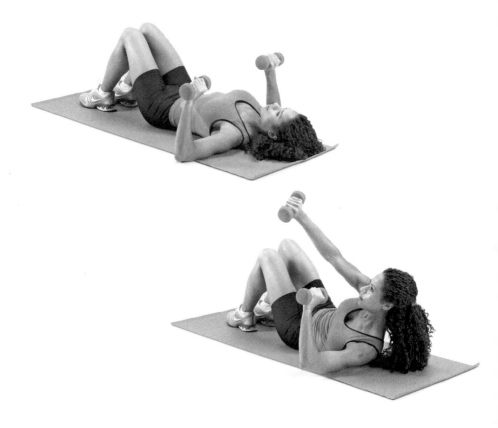

MAKE IT EASIER: Perform the move without weights.

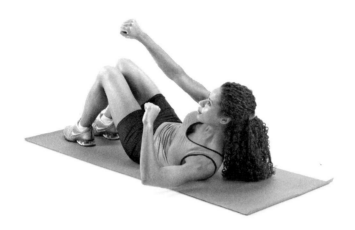

MAKE IT HARDER: Punch to each side before lowering back to the starting position.

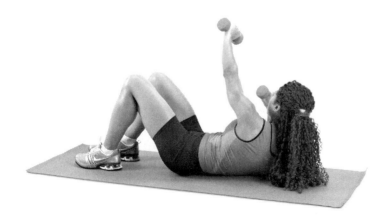

Get Your Heart Pumping: Active Calorie Cardio

Your goal is to get out of your chair and get your heart pumping a little harder for at least 30 minutes a day. You can walk, jog, swim, ride a bike, go dancing, or do whatever strikes your fancy. You don't need to huff and puff, but you should be breathing a little heavier and feeling that you're working.

As your fitness improves and you get more comfortable with your 30 minutes of movement, you can shake things up by including little bursts of higher-intensity exercise. For instance, if you usually walk, try jogging for 30 seconds. Or if you swim, pick up the pace for 10 to 25 yards. You'll not only burn more calories and get fitter faster but also beat boredom.

It's All about Flexibility: Active Calorie Stretching

A big part of Active Calorie living is movement. I want you to use your body as much as possible in every possible way. The stronger and more limber you are, the easier activity will be. As a complement to the strengthening moves, I have provided some easy daily stretches. These flexibility moves are designed to give you a full-body stretch, especially targeting common tight spots in your hamstrings, inner thighs, calves, back, and shoulders.

Stretching doesn't just feel good; it's also good for you. By increasing your range of motion, you can relieve back, joint, and muscle pain. It reduces stiffness, relieves stress, and can even boost your mood. For the best results, do these stretches most days of the week (every day, if possible), preferably when your muscles are warm, such as after a walk or an exercise session. If you stretch "cold" (meaning without some physical activity first to warm the muscles), move into the stretch more slowly and gently.

butterfly

STRETCHES: Inner thighs

1. Sit on the floor with your back straight, legs bent in front of you, and knees falling out to the sides, with the soles of your feet touching. Grasp your ankles with your hands.

2. Keeping your back straight, gently bend forward from the hips as you press your knees down toward the floor as far as comfortably possible. Hold for 20 to 30 seconds.

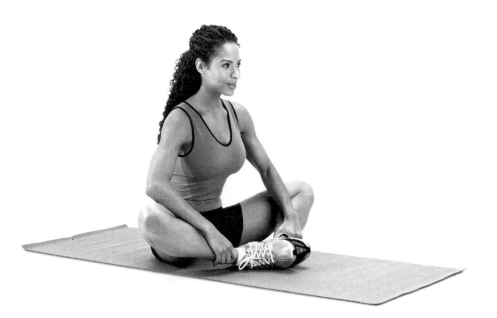

downward-facing dog

STRETCHES: Hamstrings, glutes, and calves

1. Position yourself on the floor on your hands and knees, with your feet flexed. Press your hands and feet into the floor, raising your hips toward the ceiling. Your body should look like an upside-down V.

2. Keep lifting your tailbone toward the ceiling as you lower your heels to the floor as far as comfortably possible. Hold for 20 to 30 seconds.

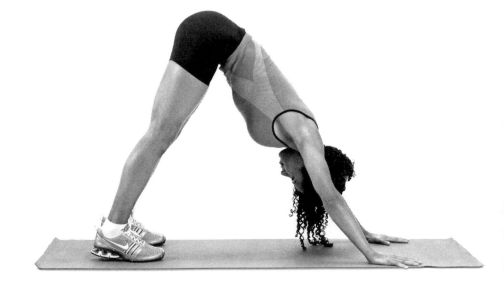

tabletop stretch

STRETCHES: Back and shoulders

1. Stand a few feet away from a sturdy chair, table, or countertop, with your feet shoulder-width apart. Lean forward slightly and grasp the chair back or place both of your palms flat on the tabletop, positioned slightly wider than shoulder-width apart. Bend your knees slightly for support.

2. Keeping your back straight and shoulders down, bend forward at the waist until your arms and back are parallel to the floor. Push your head and chest gently toward the ground until you feel a stretch. Hold, then slowly return to the starting position.

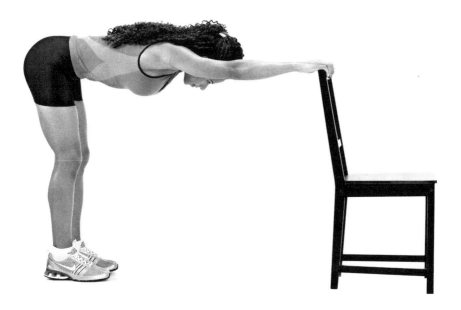

figure 4 stretch

STRETCHES: Glutes and lower back

1. Lie on your back, lift your knees toward your chest, and cross your right leg over the left so that your right ankle rests above the left knee and your right knee points out to the side.

2. Grasp behind your left leg with both hands and pull your legs closer to your body as far as comfortably possible. Hold for 15 seconds, then switch sides.

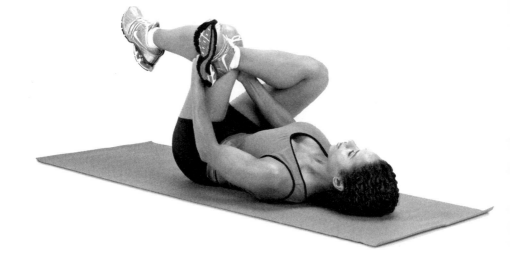

wall stretch

STRETCHES: Calves

1. Stand arm's length from a wall and place your palms flat against it. Extend your right leg behind you about 2 to 3 feet and press your right heel to the floor. (Your left knee will bend naturally as you extend back.)

2. Keep both heels flat against the floor. Hold for 15 seconds. Repeat with the opposite leg.

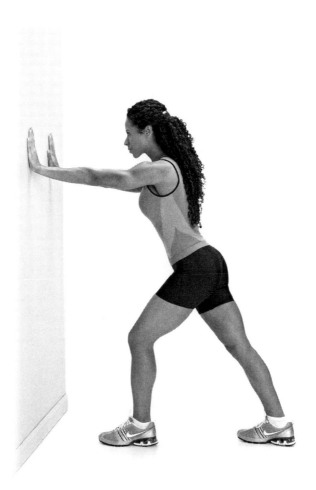

Active Life Habits

Finally, activity is not just about "exercise." It's about moving your body more all day long. The Active Calorie strength-training and cardio routines provided here are not a means to an end (that is, to a specific number of pounds lost or clothing size). They are a means to movement—to give you the strength and stamina to carry that moving momentum from your first sip of coffee to your evening cup of tea. This type of light activity is essential, whether you're a card-carrying couch potato or a marathon runner. A growing body of evidence finds that too much sitting harms your heart health. Worse, that damage is not easily undone by jumping on the elliptical trainer for 30 minutes in the morning if you spend the other 18 hours of your day planted on your rear end. A recent study of 1,579 people found that people whose jobs require more than 6 hours of chair time a day are 68 percent more likely to wind up overweight than those who sit less.[6] University of North Carolina–Wilmington researchers discovered that, on average, 68 percent of people gained weight—a lot of weight, nearly 16 pounds—within 8 months of starting a sedentary office job.[7] And in a joint effort, scientists from the University of South Carolina and Pennington Biomedical Research Center in Baton Rouge, Louisiana, found that men who spent more than 23 hours a week watching TV and sitting in cars had a 64 percent greater chance of dying from heart disease than those who sat for 11 hours a week or less, regardless of how active they were otherwise.[8] That's right: Even regular purposeful exercise wasn't enough to counteract the ill effects of so much sitting.

The solution: Stand more. By using the tips in Chapter 6, you'll be in motion more in your kitchen, the grocery store, and your garden, all day long. That alone could be enough to help you shed stubborn pounds for good. In a groundbreaking study, Mayo Clinic researchers used space-age motion-monitoring undergarments to document every fidget of 20 men and women (half lean and half obese) for 10 days. When they downloaded the data, the results were striking. Though none of the volunteers did regular structured exercise and they all held sedentary jobs, the lean men and women were in motion (standing, strolling, puttering about) 150 more minutes each day than the obese men and women, who spent that time parked in their seats.[9] The completely sedentary people burned up to 350 fewer calories each day—enough to add a pound every 10 days—just by failing to get out of their seats and on their feet! Another plus for simple lifestyle activity: It burns hundreds of calories without leaving you feeling that you need a food "reward," the way vigorous exercise sometimes does. In one study, researchers from the University of Massachusetts–Amherst measured the energy expenditure of a group of volunteers who spent literally all day sitting. If they needed to go somewhere, including the restroom, they used a wheelchair. Then the researchers took the same group and had them stand all day. They didn't do anything special—just worked on their computers and carried on as they normally would, except standing—and measured their energy expenditure for that day. The difference between sitting and standing was literally hundreds of calories (300-plus).[10]

Getting off the sofa or out of your chair is the first step. Here are other tips for moving more, even if you're stuck in an office answering phones most of the day. As I recommended in Chapter 5, you should try to incorporate these Active Life Habits as often as you can, trying at least one a day for the 4 weeks of the Active Calorie Diet.

Limit yourself to one show: Watching TV is a great way to unwind. But when it comes to the tube, there's such a thing as too much downtime. The average American tunes in for 3 hours a day, which is really bad news for your waistline, especially when you consider that watching TV burns only slightly more calories than sleeping. Harvard researchers have found that every 2 hours spent watching television increases the likelihood of obesity by 23 percent and raises your risk of developing diabetes by 14 percent. Trade 1 hour of TV time for one long walk, and you can slash your obesity risk by 24 percent and lower your risk of diabetes by 34 percent. Even just tinkering around the house for a couple of hours in the evening can lower diabetes risk by 12 percent.[11]

Can't watch just one show? Then make TV time more active by doing small tasks during commercial breaks. Pop up to take out the trash, do

SITTING STRETCHES

IF YOU WORK IN AN OFFICE, wring out your muscles twice a day and nudge your metabolism in the right direction by performing some desk stretches. These moves will also help improve your posture and help eliminate the stiff, achy shoulder, neck, and back muscles that are so common among desk jockeys.

rag doll

STRETCHES: BACK AND SHOULDERS

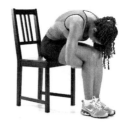

1. Sit on the edge of a chair and slump your body forward over your legs so that your chest rests on your knees and your arms hang down.
2. Wrap your arms under your knees and press your back toward the ceiling (your chest will lift off your legs). Hold for 10 seconds.

de-huncher

STRETCHES: CHEST, SHOULDERS, AND UPPER BACK

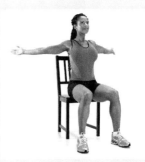

1. Sit on the edge of a chair with your legs open and your pelvis tilted slightly forward. Lift your chest and squeeze your shoulder blades together and down, away from your ears.
2. Extend your arms out from your body at 45-degree angles and reach them slightly behind you, with your palms facing forward. Hold for 10 seconds.

spinal twist

STRETCHES: BACK, SHOULDERS, AND SIDES

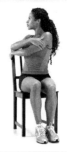

1. Sit up tall in a chair, with your feet flat on the floor. Place your right hand across your body on your left upper arm.
2. Reach your left arm across your chest, and immediately twist to the right and grasp the back of the chair with your left hand, bringing your chin over your right shoulder as you turn. Hold for 15 seconds. Switch sides.

laundry, and clean up the kitchen. You can sneak in 14 to 24 minutes of activity during 1 hour of prime-time TV. You can even hit the floor and stretch while you watch. Also consider investing in a TiVo unit or other digital video recorder, which allows you to zap through the commercials and watch many of your favorite shows in nearly half the time.

Take the stairs: There's a reason an exercise machine called the Stair-Master exists: Taking the stairs is really good exercise! In one study, exercise scientists calculated that by taking just two more flights of stairs (up and down) each day, you could burn off 6 pounds in a year.[12] Find excuses to make multiple trips between floors at work (using a restroom on another floor is one way) and at home.

Think on your feet: When you're stuck for ideas at work, get up and walk the halls. Stand and stretch during phone calls. Twice a day, get up and walk to talk to a colleague instead of e-mailing. Stanford University researchers calculated that if you were to walk across your office building and back to talk to a co-worker instead of spending the same 2 minutes e-mailing, you could spare yourself 11 pounds over 10 years—effectively avoiding the "midlife spread."[13]

Take a stand: Here's my favorite cheer: "Get off the chair and on the floor; we don't want those butts/guts/thighs no more!" In that spirit, here's a very simple move that every office worker can do: Stand up. Sitting at your desk for an hour burns 63 calories. Standing burns 127, twice as many. If you have a cordless phone, you might even be able to pace a bit, just to get the blood flowing even more. Many workplaces are now offering drafting-style tables and high chairs for office workers, which gives you the option of working on your feet most of the day and sitting down to take breaks (instead of the other way around—standing when you need a break). Ask your human resources manager about them. You'll be surprised how much more energy you have when you spend your day on your feet rather than in your seat.

Get on the ball: Sit on a large stability or Swiss ball while checking e-mail in the evening. It's an easy way to engage all of your muscles for 15 to 20 minutes. You might even be inspired to do a few stretches and crunches after you log off.

Call off the household services: All those services that you hire to make your life easier can also end up making you heavier. Small daily tasks, like weeding the garden, mowing the lawn, trimming hedges, and cleaning house, can add up to an aerobic workout. In a 2-year study of 230 overweight and inactive men and women, researchers at the Cooper Institute, an aerobics-research organization in Dallas, found that those who spent 30 minutes a day raking the lawn, taking the stairs, and walking from far spaces in parking lots achieved the same improvements in fitness, blood pressure, and body fat as those who went to the gym for vigorous exercise 20 to 60 minutes at a time, 5 days a week.[14]

Embrace cooking: I'll say it again: Cooking is the best way to lose weight. Slicing, dicing, and braising burns twice as many calories as calling Jade Garden and messing around on Facebook waiting for the wontons to come. Since you're in charge of the ingredients, the food will be chock-full of Active Calories, too. Limit takeout and delivery to two meals a week, tops.

Get off the bench: If you have kids, there's no getting around soccer (or insert any sport of your choice) practice and games. But that doesn't mean you have to be a bleacher warmer. Instead of planting yourself on the sidelines for an hour or two, use the time to walk around the field. Or volunteer to help carry equipment and assist the coach.

Park 'n' walk: It's no surprise that during the past 20 years, the number of miles we travel per day by car correlates with the rise in the number of people who are now overweight. We drive far too much and walk far too little, and it's packing on unprecedented weight around our waistlines. One of the fastest ways to get fit is to break your driving habit. Next time you have multiple errands to run, park in one central location and do them all on foot. It may take longer than driving, but you won't have to make time to exercise later.

Make it a date: Dinner and a movie is nice, but it's at least 4 hours of sitting and eating. Expand your horizons and seek out more-active forms of entertainment. Try visiting a museum, window-shopping, or even bowling. At parties, play Pictionary or charades instead of hovering over the chips and dip.

Strike up the band: Lightweight exercise bands are ideal for any office or home setting. Tie one around the leg of your desk and perform rows and arm curls while you chat on the phone. Most bands come with a poster or booklet for even more on-the-go exercise ideas.

Consider a stepper: Office workers are ideal candidates for a portable mini stepper like the Stamina InStride Electronic Mini Stepper—essentially, just two small StairMaster-like pedals without the giant machine attached. Research from the Mayo Clinic found that workers who used these clever step devices while making phone calls or answering e-mail burned an extra 290 calories an hour—enough to burn off more than 40 pounds over the course of a year if they used the machines just 2 hours a day.[15] The strategy is a little unconventional but worth considering. The stepper is relatively inexpensive and small enough to slide under your desk when you're not using it. Stepping is also something you can do while watching TV at night.

Dance, dance, dance! Pick up a few pairs of portable iPod speakers and put them in your kitchen, laundry room, and anywhere you do routine chores. Then turn up some tunes and wiggle it while you work. Music naturally inspires you to move and jazzes up even the most mundane tasks. Keep the iPod on in the house and dance all day.

Test panelist Camilla Monti swears by this tip, especially while she's making dinner. "I dance to every crazy song on the *Grease* sound track!" she says with a laugh. "The kitchen CD player is my most reliable cooking friend."

10

Live More:
Maintaining the
Active Calorie
Lifestyle

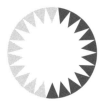

I won't lie. Losing weight, as challenging as it can be, is really the easy part. Anyone who has dropped a pant size or more before knows that keeping those lost pounds off is where the real work begins. Why is that? Many reasons. The biggest, I believe, is that too often, people look at the changes they made to lose the weight in the first place as temporary. They have a notion that those pounds are like an unwanted overcoat. Once they take the pounds off, they can resume living as they did before, and the pounds will effortlessly stay off. Another is what I call reward creep. People start rewarding their weight loss and new figure with food. I had a client say to me just the other day, "Once I lose those 10 pounds, I somehow start thinking, *I'm a skinny person now. I can eat that pumpkin cupcake because I'm not watching my weight anymore.*" Admit it: You've probably succumbed to this type of delusion yourself. We all have at one point or another. My hope is that through the Active Calorie plan, you've learned to approach food differently—that this hasn't been a diet but a change in your relationship with food.

I also hope that this has become a true lifestyle change. Every step of the Active Calorie plan has been carefully crafted to make you more physically, mentally, and metabolically active. That's a change that should stick. If it does, weight loss will stick. In a study presented at the

National Association for the Study of Obesity, researchers found that those who were overweight and hadn't changed their habits took significantly fewer steps (5,000, to be exact) than their thinner peers who had adopted Active Calorie–type lifestyle changes and regularly took 11,000 steps a day.[1] That difference in daily activity level is enough to keep nearly any stubborn pounds at bay for the better part of your days. Here's a look at the other essentials of Active Calorie living and how it will help you maintain weight loss long term.

Think Before You Eat

Journaling is an essential component of the Active Calorie plan. In the journal section starting on page 268, I've given you space to record not only what you eat but also how you feel before and after. Then I ask you to record your thoughts, observations, and challenges as you progress through the plan. This isn't to torture you, though some of my clients have likened it to medieval practices. It is to make you more aware of why you eat what you eat and how that makes you feel. This level of self-knowledge is a huge factor in long-term success—or lack thereof.

Some of the volunteers on the test panel knew their triggers. They ate chips when they were bored or frustrated and ice cream at the end of the day when fatigue set in. Others had some important revelations. "Just driving up the driveway at my mom's house triggered the desire to eat," noted one panelist. "Journaling made me aware of just how much I ate in those situations." That's precisely the awakening that I hope you have. You'll never be able to completely avoid those moods that make you want to dive into a bag of Dove bars. You can't avoid your mom forever, even if you want to (and I sincerely hope you do not). But if you recognize a craving for what it is—just an urge brought on not by hunger but by something outside your stomach—you are better equipped to quell it with something equally satisfying but nowhere nearly as fattening. It's that empowerment that can help you stay lean for life.

In a recent study of a group of women who maintained a loss of 15 to 144 pounds for at least 1 year and as long as 27 years, Yale researchers found that the successful women moved through a very specific pattern of behavior en route to permanent change.[2] When they started, the women were unaware of what contributed to their weight gain. Once they decided to make a change, they took control, learned their triggers and self-destructive behaviors, and actively began to change their responses to those triggers and stop those behaviors. Finally, after quite a few backslides, they moved into a stage of self-confidence, where they knew the behaviors they needed to change, believed that they could change them, and did change once and for all. This is not to say that you'll never again be tempted to polish off a plate of cookies because you're feeling blue. But so long as you stay in touch with your feelings, you'll be more likely to stop at one or two (okay, maybe three) cookies and channel your behavior in a more productive (and slimming) direction.

What are those more productive directions? Actions rather than reactions. Instead of eating and overeating, long-term "losers" take a walk around the block, go for a bike ride, call or e-mail a friend, update their résumé, or take other concrete actions that make them feel better—not just in the moment but for the foreseeable future. Very often the simplest way to stop unwanted eating before it starts is to simply ask "Why am I eating this?" Your answer will point you in the right direction.

Rank Your Hunger

Part of being an active eater is being aware of your food needs and how you feel. So many of us just eat on cue (e.g., It's noon; time for lunch) and keep on eating until the food is gone, regardless of whether we were really hungry when we began or started feeling full halfway through the meal. I want you to rank your hunger when you first sit down to eat and then again when you're done.

"The hunger-rating system really helps me measure and estimate my current state of hunger and fullness level," says Natalie Wingard, who lost more than 7 inches in just 4 weeks. "It's an excellent measurement tool I can use to gauge when I should be eating and when I'm just eating impulsively because I feel like it." Natalie also told me how using the scale made her conscious of eating more slowly, which definitely made her feel full sooner.

Rank hunger and fullness on the following scales.

HUNGER WHEN YOU SIT DOWN TO A MEAL

1: Satisfied. Not hungry at all

3: Comfortable. Not thinking about food, but you could eat

5: Ravenous. So hungry you could eat the legs off the chair

FULLNESS WHEN YOU ARE DONE EATING

1: Hungry. Feels like you didn't even eat

3: Satisfied. Comfortably full

5: Stuffed. One more bite, and food shoots out of your nostrils

Ideally, you'll start at a 3 on the hunger scale. Pay close attention to how you're feeling as you eat. When you reach the 3 on the fullness scale, it's time to put down your fork and stop eating.

Enlist Support

Research shows that we gain weight the same way we party: We tend to do it more in the company of others. When we hang out with people who love nachos and a few beers and grab ice cream after a big dinner, we do the same. Married people gain more weight than single people. If you have heavy friends, you're more likely to pack on some pounds, too. Well, the reverse is also true. You're more likely to lose weight and keep it off if you surround yourself with people who have similar goals.

Straight out of the gate, I got this e-mail from Camilla Monti, a test panelist who dropped a size during her first month on the plan. "Starting this week, Jeannette and I are going to COT [Cook on Thursdays] after work for the next 4 weeks. We decided on our lunch-hour walk (to Subway) today that we will prepare our culinary delights for the following many days! We're very excited and ultrapositive! I invited Carole, Michelle, and Kimberly to join us too . . . still waiting to hear back from the other gal palz :-)." I knew right there and then that Camilla would be successful. She, like many women, travels in social circles that are a huge part of her life and her happiness. To leave those circles would make her unhappy. So she decided to bring them along for the ride! And guess what? They lost weight, too.

That's the power of social support. Studies show that among people who have never been overweight, as well as those who have maintained weight loss, about 75 percent rely heavily on social support to stay on track. Among those who have lost and regained weight, only 38 percent reported using social support.[3] The more social support you have, the better your results. Turn a friend (or two) on to Active Calorie eating. Get your spouse involved. Take cooking classes together. Join a dance class. Make it fun. Keep it social. When you're all in it together, you're all far more likely to succeed.

Accentuate the Positive

I've seen it time and time again. Clients have one bad moment with a Boston cream doughnut, and before you know it, they've decided that they've "blown it," so they might as well have another slice of sausage pizza at dinner and a bag of buttery popcorn in front of the tube later that night. Why? Why? Why? Because we have this awful tendency to focus on the negative and let one slip take us down a slippery slope to dietary disaster. Enough, already!

You are going to eat some Couch Potato Calories. Get over it. Move on. Don't let that define you. Instead, focus on all the good Active Calorie foods you've eaten. Good choices beget good choices. As one of my clients put it, "Making good choices early in the day makes it easier to keep making good choices." Likewise, if you remind yourself how far you've come and all the smart meals you've eaten, you'll see that they outweigh the less-than-healthy fare. That's what to focus on. When you slip up and eat more Couch Potato Calories than you should, just get right back on the path and make sure the next few meals and snacks are active. It's all just a balancing act. So keep your eyes forward, and don't let one little slipup sidetrack all the hard work you've done. With time this, too, will become automatic.

Burn, Baby, Burn

I've said it before; I'll say it again. If you want to keep off the weight, you have to exercise. A tall and growing body of research shows that burning calories through exercise is more important for weight loss maintenance than losing the weight in the first place. When the National Weight Control Registry examined the exercise habits of more than 3,600 men and women who had managed to keep off at least 30 pounds for at least a year, exercise was a key habit, with the participants doing the equivalent of either 60 to 75 minutes a day of moderate activity, like brisk walking, or 35 to 45 minutes a day of more intense exercise, like running or cycling.

Another way to look at the activity level you need to maintain weight loss is to consider calories burned each week. Research shows that dieters who remain slender burn about 2,800 calories per week, or 400 calories per day, through exercise. Sounds like a lot. But once you get moving, it adds up fast. As you sit there flipping pages, you burn about one calorie per minute. That number jumps each time you stand, walk, or run to pick up the phone because your body needs more energy to get the job done. The more muscles you move and/or the harder you work, the more calories you will burn. Here are the calorie-burning rates of some popular sporting activities. (They're based on a 140-pound woman. If you're heavier, you'll burn more; lighter, you'll burn less.)

CALORIE INCINERATORS: 600-PLUS CALORIES AN HOUR

Running (moderate, 10-minute miles)

Trail running

Road biking (fast, 16 mph)

Swimming the breaststroke

Karate (or other martial arts)

Jumping rope (moderate to fast)

Soccer, competitive

Inline skating

Step aerobics (with a high, 10-inch step)

BIG BURNERS: 400 TO 500-PLUS CALORIES AN HOUR

Rowing (moderate to hard)

Tennis

Swimming freestyle, easy

Elliptical training

Day hiking (local trails with a pack)

Circuit training (hard, with some vigorous cardio between sets)

Cross-country skiing, easy pace (use a machine when there's no snow)

Spinning

Cardio dance class (e.g., funk)

STEADY SCORCHERS: 300 TO 400 AN HOUR

Kayaking

African dancing

Weight lifting (dumbbells and Nautilus)

Power walking (4.0 to 4.5 mph)

Hiking without a pack

Body-sculpting class

Low-impact cardio class

Jazz dance

Walk-jog intervals

EASY SIMMERS: 200 TO 300 AN HOUR

Flamenco, belly, or swing dancing

Pilates (general mat work)

Brisk walking (3.5 mph)

Yoga (flowing)

Golfing (carrying clubs)

Water aerobics

Tai chi

Abs class

When you look at that list, there's really no excuse not to burn the calories you need to keep the weight off. Mix and match, and find a few activities that you love and will do for life. The more you do, the more successful (and, I'd venture to say, the happier) you'll be.

Create an Energy Gap

Here's the unfair truth: Because your calorie-burning metabolism is largely based on your size, once you drop pounds, you need fewer calories than you did before you lost the weight. If you've lost 10 to 15 percent of your body weight—or about 20 to 30 pounds for someone who started at 180—you'll need 200 to 300 fewer calories a day to maintain your new trim weight and keep the pounds from coming back.

This is yet another reason that exercise is essential in maintaining weight loss. Yes, you could slash your food intake by another couple hundred calories—the amount in a banana and yogurt—every day. But let's face it: That starts to feel a lot like deprivation. Isn't it far more fun to enroll in a dance class, take a bike ride, or play a round of golf? Absolutely! Is your schedule just too packed to fit in more activity on a given day? Then go half and half. Trim your daily calorie intake by about 150 calories, or the amount in an English muffin, and sneak in three quick 10- to 15-minute walks to fill in the gap.

Cull the Closet

I have a client who has been struggling with the same 10 pounds for about as many years. She's not thrilled with the situation, but she is happy that her regain has never pushed past the 10-pound mark. Her secret: "I never buy new pants." She can fit into most of her wardrobe within that 10-pound range. Once she creeps further into the double-digit weight gain, she's in danger of wearing clothes from the famed emperor's closet because there's nothing left that will fit.

To me this is a crucial form of accountability. Once you've lost weight, bag up your heavy clothes and send them packing to the Salvation Army. Invest in some stylish outfits in your new, smaller size that make you look as good as you feel. Too many of my clients own a full wardrobe in about six different sizes. That makes it far too easy to toss accountability out the window and yo-yo up and down on the scale.

Weigh In

There are plenty of dietitians who will advise you to eschew the scale. I'm not one of them. It's not that I'm in favor of people maniacally obsessing over every single pound. I most definitely am not. But there's just too much strong evidence that suggests that weighing yourself periodically is one of the single best ways to maintain weight loss. The why is simple: You can see the pounds creeping back on—and do something about it—before the situation gets out of control.

Such consistent self-monitoring is one of the hallmarks of the successful long-term "losers" in the National Weight Control Registry. How often should you weigh yourself? Many of the registry participants weigh in daily. That feels like a bit too much for me. Your weight naturally goes up and down a few pounds as you lose and retain water (especially women), so you have the potential to drive yourself bananas. Weekly feels about right. I like Monday morning, right after you wake up and use the bathroom but before you eat. Track your Monday-morning weight. If it creeps up by 3 pounds or more, pull in the reins on your Couch Potato Calories and/or pick up your activity level.

Like tossing your old "overweight" clothes, regular weighing sends a signal to your brain that you're serious about this and committed for the long haul. That commitment will spill over and help you make smart Active Calorie decisions during the day because you know you're accountable to yourself. Some women have such a strong negative reaction to the scale that this step is difficult. But remember this: No one—*no one*—but you has to know what that number is. Heck, you

TRIED-AND-TRUE TIPS FOR KEEPING IT OFF

THE NATIONAL WEIGHT CONTROL REGISTRY keeps track of thousands of individuals who have lost weight and kept it off. Here are the top weight-maintenance strategies among those who lost more than 60 pounds and kept it off for at least 2 years.

- Eat breakfast regularly. Most eat a morning meal every single day.

- Step on the scale. Successful losers monitor their weight regularly, often daily (though I think weekly is fine).

- Burn about 400 calories every day through exercise—about an hour's worth a day.

- Walk the walk. Most of them take many steps every day—some studies suggest that 11,000 is the magic number.

- Control portions and calorie intake. The Active Calorie plan makes that a no-brainer!

can lie (not to yourself, of course) if you want. But not knowing the number isn't going to change what it is. And ultimately it doesn't matter what that actual number is. It matters that the number stays put and doesn't keep going up. The only way you'll really know this is to step on the scale.

Befriend Breakfast

I feel as if I've repeated this more times than a *Seinfeld* rerun, but it's so important that it bears mentioning yet again! Nearly 80 percent of the nearly 3,000 participants in the National Weight Control Registry eat breakfast 7 days a week. Again, that morning meal does not have to be elaborate, but it's important that it exists because it sets the stage for long-term success.

{ natalie wingard }

Forging a New Relationship with Food

AGE: 42

POUNDS LOST:

5.6

INCHES LOST:

7½ Including 3 off her waist

NATALIE WINGARD had always been fairly active and healthy, but she never thought much about food. In fact, she often skipped breakfast entirely. Now she has fully embraced the Active Calorie lifestyle, from choosing to prepping to fully enjoying her food. She can barely believe the difference in her energy and satisfaction.

"I use all fresh ingredients and use as much activity to prepare the meals so I keep my system moving and burning calories. For example, I always use block cheese and grate it. This one extra small step keeps me moving more vigorously while preparing my meal. I absolutely love the breakfast burrito. It's spicy and flavorful and a very satisfying meal emotionally. I love how it causes my body temperature to rise and my sinuses to open as I break a bit of a sweat. The heat also helps me slow down between bites, which helps me not overeat. I notice I have much more energy walking to work in the morning."

Natalie has taken the Active Calorie approach one extra step by growing her own food! "I do something active in my herb and vegetable garden every day," she says, noting that by watering, weeding, and doing the general upkeep of her garden, she gets more exercise, too.

There are 16 breakfast options to choose from in Chapter 7, starting on page 106. If you haven't yet (and I really hope you have), try some. See how it feels to eat a little more in the morning. I'm betting that you'll be happier, more energetic, and more satisfied all day long.

Frequently Asked Questions

The benefit of doing a test run with a panel of real men and women is that I can pinpoint the trouble spots, see what people like (and what they don't), and generally work out the kinks for a smooth-running plan that I hope will please most people. That said, you're still bound to have a query or two as you ease your way into Active Calorie living. Here are the answers to questions I'm asked most often.

Q. **I find that I have developed some bloating and irregularity since starting the Active Calorie meal plan. Should I pick up some Beano or probiotics to see if they take care of the problem?**

A: If you weren't eating much fiber in your diet before and you suddenly make a big increase with lots of fiber-rich fruits and vegetables, you might run into some bloating issues as your gastrointestinal system adjusts. First and foremost, follow the Active Calorie recommendation to drink 2 cups of water before and with meals. It will help your body break down the fiber and flush your digestive system so you avoid constipation, which can cause bloating. Rinse beans before you eat them in order to reduce the bloat-causing starch. Eat slowly, thoroughly chewing your food. Staying active, like taking a walk after dinner, also helps stimulate digestion and keeps you from feeling bloated and sluggish. If you do still want to take Beano, do so before eating. I don't recommend probiotics as part of the Active Calorie Diet. By eating more veggies and including some yogurt in your diet, you get all the probiotics you need naturally.

Q: **. I have to work 2 or 3 nights a week, so food preparation is
. challenging. Any advice for making it easier?**

A: Believe me, I understand! I spent more than 1 evening a week
burning a little midnight oil when writing this book. Though it's
great to cook dinner fresh when possible, freezing is a fabulous
option for having a great Active Calorie meal ready to go in minutes
when it's not. You'll notice that many of the recipes offered in
Chapter 7 make four or more servings. If you know that you don't
have time during the week, make a little extra one night (I like
Sunday for doing this) and freeze the rest. In fact, if you find yourself with some spare time during the weekend, you can cook up a
few dishes to freeze. That way you'll always have something healthy
and handy to eat when life gets in the way!

Q: **. I'm finding the plan a challenge because I am on the road
. most of the time as part of my job. I never know where I will
be or when I will get to eat. That leaves me pretty vulnerable to
the boxes of doughnuts my co-workers bring in. What can I do?**

A: I understand being on the road! It's a huge hurdle for even the
most health-conscious eater to overcome. But you can make the
Active Calorie plan work on the go. It just takes a little forethought.
I would recommend having a few Active Calorie snacks in your
truck or car to help you avoid temptation when hunger calls. Try
keeping a pack of jerky, some nuts, and some bananas on board to
grab and eat when you have to go more than a few hours between
meals. You can pick up an insulated lunch bag at Walmart or Target
to have even more options on hand. In it you can keep perishable
fruit, yogurt, hard-cooked eggs, packets of tuna, whole wheat
crackers, string cheese, baby carrots, and V8. And try Crystal Light
packs that you can mix with water to give you something flavorful
to stay hydrated during those long hours on the road.

When you are simply stuck out there with no snacks available, check out the healthy fast-food choices in Chapter 8. Subway is always an option. Wendy's has healthy chili. Even McDonald's Egg McMuffins aren't so bad when you need to eat on the run. Once you see all the Active Calorie choices available, you'll find that eating on the road can be smooth sailing. Finally, if the boredom of being confined in a car is what is drawing you to those Munchkins, keep a pack of gum handy at all times and pop a piece to keep your mouth fresh and busy—and help you avoid sugary sweets or salty snacks.

Q: **I am terrible with food selection in high-risk situations, like parties, baseball games, and picnics. How can I enjoy myself and stay on the plan, too?**

A: You can't live life without ball games, parties, and picnics! But you can have fun while still losing fat. I won't lie. There are some sacrifices involved. But with smart planning, they can be small ones. First, don't go to these functions hungry. Eat a filling but not calorie-dense Active Calorie snack, such as an apple or some baby carrots—and drink a 16-ounce bottle of water before you go. It'll be just enough to fill you up a little so that you're not easily swayed by the goodies you don't really want. (If you show up to a ball game ravenous, you're likely to plow through a bag of even the stalest popcorn.)

When you get where you're going, take some time to survey the food available and choose the one thing that really appeals to you. Help yourself to one serving of it, and then fill your plate with Active Calorie options—fruit, a green salad, and so forth. And remember that Active Calorie foods include many of your favorite snacks and foods. (See page 212 for some good choices.) The idea is to satisfy your yearning for the Couch Potato picnic or party fare while also filling yourself up on plenty of good stuff so that you're simply too full to overdo it. Remember, Active Calorie living is not all or nothing. It's not about feeling constantly deprived. It's looking at food through a new lens, making smart, more active choices one meal, snack, party, and ball game at a time.

Q. **Should I take a vitamin-mineral supplement while on this program?**

A: The role of a supplement is to support health, not to replace food. I strongly believe in food first. That being said, when you are watching portion sizes, you may not always get every vitamin and mineral from your meals, especially if you are a vegetarian or have food allergies or sensitivities, so you may want to add a supplement.

Look for products with the United States Pharmacopeia (USP) symbol, which verifies that the product contains what it should and is free of contaminants, and read the label and follow the dosage instructions. Some prescription and over-the-counter medications do not mix well with supplements.

Congratulations on completing the Active Calorie Diet. You may not realize it now, but you've hopped on the first wave of a sea change in how people think about the food they eat. As we were finishing this manuscript, the news broke that Weight Watchers was changing its points system for the first time in a decade and a half. Why? I quote:

"It's a complete overhaul; it doesn't get any bigger than this," said Karen Miller-Kovach, the chief scientific officer for Weight Watchers International. "Fifteen years ago we said a calorie is a calorie is a calorie. If you ate 100 calories of butter or 100 calories of chicken, it was all the same. Now, we know that is not the case in terms of how hard the body has to work to make that energy available. And even more important is that where that energy comes from affects feelings of hunger and fullness."

THE ACTIVE CALORIE DIET AT A GLANCE

FOLLOW THESE SIMPLE GUIDELINES to activate every calorie—and your life!

- Eat three meals (breakfast, lunch, and dinner) and a snack every day.

- Make sure each meal follows the Active Calorie Plate proportions (snacks and desserts may have only one type of Active Calorie): a little more than a quarter should be chewy protein; about half should be chewy and hearty fruits and vegetables; a little less than a quarter should be hearty grains.

- Have at least one energizing food—such as coffee, tea, and dark chocolate—or warming food—such as chile pepper, cinnamon, garlic, and ginger—per meal (not including snacks). See page 67 for the complete list.

- Drink two glasses of water with every meal.

- Do at least one Active Eating Habit (see Chapter 6) and one Active Life Habit (see Chapter 9) every day.

Sound familiar? It sure did to us. We're thrilled to be on the cutting edge of calorie science. And we're proud to be able to explain to you which calories are most active, which are complete Couch Potatoes, and even how to transform some of those lazy calories so you don't have to completely dismiss them from your diet. Even better, we are giving you dozens of recipes, meal plans, and journal pages to get you on the right path. All you have to do is follow the diet for 4 weeks and it will become automatic. You'll know what good, Active Calorie food looks, feels, and tastes like. And, more importantly, how it makes you feel.

In just 4 weeks we saw the 17 women and men on our test panel transform their bodies, shapes, and skin. We saw them finally be able to ditch their meds. We saw whole families transform in front of our eyes. They got healthier, leaner, more active, and happier. Now, it's your turn. I wish you the best of health.

Appendix A

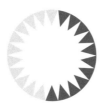

The Active Calorie Diet Journal

Being accountable to someone is a huge component of weight loss success. That's why groups like Weight Watchers are so successful. You know you have to weigh in and answer to the group each week. That's fine for the short term, but ultimately you need to learn how to be accountable to yourself. That's where journaling comes in. By writing down every meal and snack, you'll not only spot trends and food triggers but also feel a sense of commitment and accountability.

But I don't want you to become a fanatic about writing down every last calorie. The goal is awareness of your daily activity level and food habits. I want you to discover the sedentary spots in your routine and find places where you can "activate" your day by moving around. And I want you to take some time on the weekends to review your progress, consider which changes are working best, and make a plan for the coming week. As you fill in the blanks on these journal pages, you'll be forging new healthful habits—and leaving behind the old.

I've provided a week's worth of blank pages for a daily journal and a weekly review here. You can photocopy them to use as often as you'd like, or you can buy *The Active Calorie Diet Journal*—which gives you the space to track your Active Calories (and your active life!) for up to 12 weeks—at www.prevention.com/shop, or call 800-848-4735.

Most of the information required in the following journal pages is pretty self-explanatory. After taking a look at the sample pages we've provided, you'll probably have no trouble making them work for you. However, there are a few details I should discuss before you get started.

Learn to Rank Your Hunger— And Your Fullness

So many people eat on cue, and keep eating until the food is gone, that they lose track of whether they were really hungry to begin with or started feeling full halfway through the meal. That's why my rating system asks you to rank your hunger when you first sit down to eat *and* your fullness when you're done. Use it to gauge when you should be eating and when you're eating impulsively. As a bonus, paying attention to your hunger will also help you eat more slowly, which definitely makes you feel full sooner.

HUNGER WHEN YOU SIT DOWN TO A MEAL

1: Satisfied. Not hungry at all

3: Comfortable. Not thinking about food, but you could eat

5: Ravenous. So hungry you could eat the legs off the chair

1: Hungry. Feels like you didn't even eat

3: Satisfied. Comfortably full

5: Stuffed. One more bite, and food shoots out of your nostrils

Ideally, you'll start at a 3 on the hunger scale. Pay close attention to how you're feeling as you eat. When you reach the 3 on the fullness scale, it's time to put down your fork and stop eating.

Keep Track of Couch Potato Calories

At the bottom of every daily entry page, you will find a space that asks you to keep track of any less-than-healthy foods you may have had. Keeping tabs on your Couch Potato Calories is in keeping with the Active Calorie Diet philosophy. I say go ahead and have that doughnut once in a while (like on a Friday). But if you pay attention to when exactly you'll have it, you'll probably be more inclined to eat it early in the day instead of late afternoon. (That's a good thing, because quick-burning carbs seem to spike insulin more when you eat them later in the day.) Of course, just because you see a space for Couch Potato foods in your journal does not mean it's a license to have a pastry every day. But once in a while, I understand, especially if you're keeping track of your treats.

Weigh Yourself Regularly

Your weight naturally goes up and down a few pounds as you lose and retain water (especially true for women), so you have the potential to drive yourself bananas if you try to weigh yourself daily. I suggest that you weigh yourself just once a week instead. Try to pick the same time each week—like Monday morning, right after you wake up and use the bathroom but before you eat. If the numbers on the scale creep up by 3 pounds or more, you'll know it's time to ramp up your Active Calories and/or pick up your activity level.

Keep Adding—and Keep Track of—Active Habits

Remember that you want to keep adding Active Eating and Active Life Habits to your day whenever possible. Here's a summary of the ideas I listed in Chapters 6 and 9 that you can try. But of course, you're not limited to these. Make up your own active habits to fuel your Active Calorie lifestyle.

ACTIVE EATING HABITS

Get (at least) one good knife.

Use nonstick pans.

Make lists.

Shop more often.

Read the labels.

Buy whole produce.

Stock up on spices.

Measure and weigh portions.

Cook veggies crunchy.

Order steak medium-rare.

Serve up a salad.

Spritz and spray cooking spray.

Steam veggies.

Go for the grill.

Slow-cook it.

Blend it.

Break away from baking.

Think outside the breading box.

Add some zest.

Peel it; press it.

Grind it up.

Rank your hunger.

Downsize your dishes (if yours are currently full size or larger).

Serve yourself restaurant style.

Serve from the stove.

Eat at the table.

Use your utensils.

Take smaller bites and chew more.

Clean the cupboards.

Put treats out of sight.

Put produce on display.

Label your spices.

Create your own grab-and-gos.

Pack lunches or snacks.

Turn off the television.

Shed light on your meals.

Put mirrors in your kitchen and dining room.

Clear the clutter in your kitchen and dining room.

Journal what you eat.

Limit TV watching.

Take the stairs.

Think on your feet.

Stand while working.

Get on a stability or Swiss ball.

Call off the household services.

Embrace cooking.

Get off the bench.

Park 'n' walk.

Make your dates active.

Try a resistance band.

Consider a stepper.

Dance, dance, dance!

Because changing your activity level is every bit as important as changing your eating style, we ask you to track how much movement you're able to accomplish every day. You'll find space to record your gym time along with new habits you're trying to adopt. But just like we ask you to keep an eye on Couch Potato Calories, you're also asked to note the inactive parts of your day. How much time was spent watching television or staring at a computer screen? Make your best estimate and see if you can bring that number down over the long haul. At the end of every week, we'll ask you to reflect on how energized you felt over the last 7 days. Rank your energy level on the following scale:

1: I'm surprised I was able to get out of bed in the morning.

3: I was able to get through the week without feeling overly tired.

5: I had more energy than a 5-year-old.

WEEK: 3

	TIME	LOCATION
BREAKFAST	8:00	home

How I'm feeling: _ambitious—_
a lot to do today

Hunger before meal: 2

Fullness after meal: 4

Liquids: ☑ ☑

Energizing or Warming Active Calories:

pinch of cayenne

Fruit and vegetable: _½ cup raspberries_

Protein: _8 oz Greek yogurt_
2 T almonds

Grain: _¾ cup bran cereal_

	TIME	LOCATION
LUNCH	10:00	park—picnic!

How I'm feeling: _glad to be_
outdoors

Hunger before meal: _____

Fullness after meal: _____

Liquids: ☑ ☐

Energizing or Warming Active Calories:

green tea

Fruit and vegetable: _grapes_
1 cup cucumber/tomato/onion
salad

Protein: _1 oz part-skim Swiss cheese_
¼ cup chickpeas in salad

Grain: _whole wheat baguette—_
small piece

	TIME	LOCATION
DINNER	7:30	Mike's Deck

How I'm feeling: _relaxed—_
evening w/friends

Hunger before meal: 3

Fullness after meal: 4

Liquids: ☑ ☑

Energizing or Warming Active Calories:

coffee; candied
ginger on pineapple

Fruit and vegetable: _grilled asparagus_
+ grilled pineapple for dessert

Protein: _4 oz grilled chicken_
breast—drizzled
with lemon juice

Grain: _½ cup quinoa_
pilaf

	TIME	LOCATION
SNACK	4:00	home

How I'm feeling: _____

Hunger before meal: _____

Fullness after meal: _____

Liquids: ☐ ☐

Energizing or Warming Active Calories:

extra splash of hot
sauce + black pepper

Fruit and vegetable: _carrot_
celery

Protein: _¼ cup blue cheese dip_

Grain: _____

CARDIO WORKOUT

ACTIVITY	DURATION	INTENSITY	LOCATION
Tennis	30 min	5	Riverview Park

STRENGTH TRAINING

EXERCISE	WEIGHTS	REPS	COMMENTS
step & extend	5	8	try 9 reps next
split squat/curl	5	12	
single leg row	4	10	
dip & crunch	—	9	
chest press punch	3	9	no second set
lateral lift	3	10	

Active Life Habits: ___TV free day! Talked on the phone__
with my sister while I picked up around the house

Active Eating Habits: ___Helped Mike with a great bbq.__
Brought dishes I could share—everyone loved the pineapple!

Time spent sitting: ___4½ hours__

Food reflections: *Use this space to record what went well (and perhaps not so well) for you today.*
having afternoon snack made late dinner easier to handle

My Week at a Glance

Starting weight: _163_

Ending weight: _155_

Total weight loss: _8 pounds (2 this week)_

ACTIVE CALORIE SUMMARY

Total number of restaurant meals: _1_

Total number of take-out meals: _4_

Total number of ready-to-eat meals: _2_

Total number of trips to the grocery store: _4_

I tried these Active Eating Habits: _made 3 dishes that I could freeze in small portions—no tempting leftovers_

I tried these Active Calorie foods: _grilled pineapple, Greek yogurt, roasted poblano, barley_

I had these Couch Potato Calorie foods: _1 glazed doughnut
1 small bag corn chips_

Thinking about the week ahead, I think my biggest challenge will be: _2 business dinners coming up—remember to review menus beforehand_

ACTIVE LIFE SUMMARY

Total time I spent exercising: _5½ hours_

My overall energy level for the week (circle one):   1   2   3   4   ⑤

Total time I spent sitting this week: _32_

I tried these Active Life Habits: _Focused on cooking when I could. Walked more at work—even had one phone meeting where I stood the whole time._

My favorite activity is: _Tennis & hiking were both great this week._

What I learned about myself:
—_planning is important to my success and saves me time in the long run_
—_focusing on being active with friends is an easy way to stay in touch_
—_I'm saving $$ by doing my own yardwork!_

—Found it hard to resist the doughnuts at work, but learned that if I chew gum during the meeting, they don't taste so good so I'm less tempted.

WEEK: ____

	TIME	LOCATION

BREAKFAST

How I'm feeling: _____

_____

Hunger before meal: _____

Fullness after meal: _____

Liquids: ☐ ☐

Energizing or Warming Active Calories:

_____

_____

_____

Fruit and vegetable: _____

_____

Protein: _____

_____

Grain: _____

_____

_____

	TIME	LOCATION

LUNCH

How I'm feeling: _____

_____

Hunger before meal: _____

Fullness after meal: _____

Liquids: ☐ ☐

Energizing or Warming Active Calories:

_____

_____

_____

Fruit and vegetable: _____

_____

Protein: _____

_____

Grain: _____

_____

_____

	TIME	LOCATION

DINNER

How I'm feeling: _____

_____

Hunger before meal: _____

Fullness after meal: _____

Liquids: ☐ ☐

Energizing or Warming Active Calories:

_____

_____

_____

Fruit and vegetable: _____

_____

Protein: _____

_____

Grain: _____

_____

_____

	TIME	LOCATION

SNACK

How I'm feeling: _____

_____

Hunger before meal: _____

Fullness after meal: _____

Liquids: ☐ ☐

Energizing or Warming Active Calories:

_____

_____

_____

Fruit and vegetable: _____

_____

Protein: _____

_____

Grain: _____

_____

_____

CARDIO WORKOUT

ACTIVITY	DURATION	INTENSITY	LOCATION

STRENGTH TRAINING

EXERCISE	WEIGHTS	REPS	COMMENTS

Active Life Habits: _____

_____

_____

Active Eating Habits: _____

_____

_____

Time spent sitting: _____

Food reflections: *Use this space to record what went well (and perhaps not so well) for you today.*

_____

_____

WEEK: ____

BREAKFAST
TIME | LOCATION

How I'm feeling: _____

Hunger before meal: _____
Fullness after meal: _____
Liquids: ☐ ☐
Energizing or Warming Active Calories:
_____
_____
_____

Fruit and vegetable: _____
_____

Protein: _____
_____

Grain: _____
_____

LUNCH
TIME | LOCATION

How I'm feeling: _____

Hunger before meal: _____
Fullness after meal: _____
Liquids: ☐ ☐
Energizing or Warming Active Calories:
_____
_____
_____

Fruit and vegetable: _____
_____

Protein: _____
_____

Grain: _____
_____

DINNER
TIME | LOCATION

How I'm feeling: _____

Hunger before meal: _____
Fullness after meal: _____
Liquids: ☐ ☐
Energizing or Warming Active Calories:
_____
_____
_____

Fruit and vegetable: _____
_____

Protein: _____
_____

Grain: _____
_____

SNACK
TIME | LOCATION

How I'm feeling: _____

Hunger before meal: _____
Fullness after meal: _____
Liquids: ☐ ☐
Energizing or Warming Active Calories:
_____
_____
_____

Fruit and vegetable: _____
_____

Protein: _____
_____

Grain: _____
_____

DAY: _____

CARDIO WORKOUT

ACTIVITY	DURATION	INTENSITY	LOCATION

STRENGTH TRAINING

EXERCISE	WEIGHTS	REPS	COMMENTS

Active Life Habits: _____

_____

_____

_____

Active Eating Habits: _____

_____

_____

_____

Time spent sitting: _____

Food reflections: *Use this space to record what went well (and perhaps not so well) for you today.*

_____

_____

WEEK: ____

| | TIME | LOCATION |

BREAKFAST

How I'm feeling: _____

Fruit and vegetable: _____

Hunger before meal: _____

Fullness after meal: _____

Protein: _____

Liquids: ☐ ☐

Energizing or Warming Active Calories:

Grain: _____

| | TIME | LOCATION |

LUNCH

How I'm feeling: _____

Fruit and vegetable: _____

Hunger before meal: _____

Fullness after meal: _____

Protein: _____

Liquids: ☐ ☐

Energizing or Warming Active Calories:

Grain: _____

| | TIME | LOCATION |

DINNER

How I'm feeling: _____

Fruit and vegetable: _____

Hunger before meal: _____

Fullness after meal: _____

Protein: _____

Liquids: ☐ ☐

Energizing or Warming Active Calories:

Grain: _____

| | TIME | LOCATION |

SNACK

How I'm feeling: _____

Fruit and vegetable: _____

Hunger before meal: _____

Fullness after meal: _____

Protein: _____

Liquids: ☐ ☐

Energizing or Warming Active Calories:

Grain: _____

CARDIO WORKOUT

ACTIVITY	DURATION	INTENSITY	LOCATION

STRENGTH TRAINING

EXERCISE	WEIGHTS	REPS	COMMENTS

Active Life Habits: _____

_____

_____

Active Eating Habits: _____

_____

_____

Time spent sitting: _____

Food reflections: *Use this space to record what went well (and perhaps not so well) for you today.*

_____

_____

WEEK: ___

	TIME	LOCATION
BREAKFAST		

How I'm feeling: _____

Hunger before meal: _____

Fullness after meal: _____

Liquids: ☐ ☐

Energizing or Warming Active Calories:

_____

Fruit and vegetable: _____

Protein: _____

Grain: _____

	TIME	LOCATION
LUNCH		

How I'm feeling: _____

Hunger before meal: _____

Fullness after meal: _____

Liquids: ☐ ☐

Energizing or Warming Active Calories:

_____

Fruit and vegetable: _____

Protein: _____

Grain: _____

	TIME	LOCATION
DINNER		

How I'm feeling: _____

Hunger before meal: _____

Fullness after meal: _____

Liquids: ☐ ☐

Energizing or Warming Active Calories:

_____

Fruit and vegetable: _____

Protein: _____

Grain: _____

	TIME	LOCATION
SNACK		

How I'm feeling: _____

Hunger before meal: _____

Fullness after meal: _____

Liquids: ☐ ☐

Energizing or Warming Active Calories:

_____

Fruit and vegetable: _____

Protein: _____

Grain: _____

DAY: _____

CARDIO WORKOUT

ACTIVITY	DURATION	INTENSITY	LOCATION

STRENGTH TRAINING

EXERCISE	WEIGHTS	REPS	COMMENTS

Active Life Habits: _____

_____

_____

Active Eating Habits: _____

_____

_____

Time spent sitting: _____

Food reflections: *Use this space to record what went well (and perhaps not so well) for you today.*

_____

_____

WEEK: ____

	TIME	LOCATION

BREAKFAST

How I'm feeling: _____

Hunger before meal: _____

Fullness after meal: _____

Liquids: ☐ ☐

Energizing or Warming Active Calories:
_____
_____
_____

Fruit and vegetable: _____
_____

Protein: _____
_____
_____

Grain: _____
_____
_____

LUNCH

| TIME | LOCATION |

How I'm feeling: _____

Hunger before meal: _____

Fullness after meal: _____

Liquids: ☐ ☐

Energizing or Warming Active Calories:
_____
_____
_____

Fruit and vegetable: _____
_____

Protein: _____
_____
_____

Grain: _____
_____
_____

DINNER

| TIME | LOCATION |

How I'm feeling: _____

Hunger before meal: _____

Fullness after meal: _____

Liquids: ☐ ☐

Energizing or Warming Active Calories:
_____
_____
_____

Fruit and vegetable: _____
_____

Protein: _____
_____
_____

Grain: _____
_____
_____

SNACK

| TIME | LOCATION |

How I'm feeling: _____

Hunger before meal: _____

Fullness after meal: _____

Liquids: ☐ ☐

Energizing or Warming Active Calories:
_____
_____
_____

Fruit and vegetable: _____
_____

Protein: _____
_____
_____

Grain: _____
_____
_____

DAY: ____

CARDIO WORKOUT

ACTIVITY	DURATION	INTENSITY	LOCATION

STRENGTH TRAINING

EXERCISE	WEIGHTS	REPS	COMMENTS

Active Life Habits: _____

_____

_____

Active Eating Habits: _____

_____

_____

Time spent sitting: _____

Food reflections: *Use this space to record what went well (and perhaps not so well) for you today.*

_____

_____

WEEK: ___

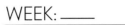

	TIME	LOCATION
BREAKFAST		

How I'm feeling: _____

_____

Hunger before meal: _____

Fullness after meal: _____

Liquids: ☐ ☐

Energizing or Warming Active Calories:

_____

_____

_____

Fruit and vegetable: _____

_____

Protein: _____

_____

Grain: _____

_____

_____

	TIME	LOCATION
LUNCH		

How I'm feeling: _____

_____

Hunger before meal: _____

Fullness after meal: _____

Liquids: ☐ ☐

Energizing or Warming Active Calories:

_____

_____

_____

Fruit and vegetable: _____

_____

Protein: _____

_____

Grain: _____

_____

_____

	TIME	LOCATION
DINNER		

How I'm feeling: _____

_____

Hunger before meal: _____

Fullness after meal: _____

Liquids: ☐ ☐

Energizing or Warming Active Calories:

_____

_____

_____

Fruit and vegetable: _____

_____

Protein: _____

_____

Grain: _____

_____

_____

	TIME	LOCATION
SNACK		

How I'm feeling: _____

_____

Hunger before meal: _____

Fullness after meal: _____

Liquids: ☐ ☐

Energizing or Warming Active Calories:

_____

_____

_____

Fruit and vegetable: _____

_____

Protein: _____

_____

Grain: _____

_____

_____

DAY: ____

CARDIO WORKOUT

ACTIVITY	DURATION	INTENSITY	LOCATION

STRENGTH TRAINING

EXERCISE	WEIGHTS	REPS	COMMENTS

Active Life Habits: _____

_____

_____

Active Eating Habits: _____

_____

_____

Time spent sitting: _____

Food reflections: *Use this space to record what went well (and perhaps not so well) for you today.*

_____

_____

WEEK: ___

BREAKFAST
TIME   LOCATION

How I'm feeling: _____

Hunger before meal: _____

Fullness after meal: _____

Liquids: ☐ ☐

Energizing or Warming Active Calories:

_____

Fruit and vegetable: _____

Protein: _____

Grain: _____

LUNCH
TIME   LOCATION

How I'm feeling: _____

Hunger before meal: _____

Fullness after meal: _____

Liquids: ☐ ☐

Energizing or Warming Active Calories:

_____

Fruit and vegetable: _____

Protein: _____

Grain: _____

DINNER
TIME   LOCATION

How I'm feeling: _____

Hunger before meal: _____

Fullness after meal: _____

Liquids: ☐ ☐

Energizing or Warming Active Calories:

_____

Fruit and vegetable: _____

Protein: _____

Grain: _____

SNACK
TIME   LOCATION

How I'm feeling: _____

Hunger before meal: _____

Fullness after meal: _____

Liquids: ☐ ☐

Energizing or Warming Active Calories:

_____

Fruit and vegetable: _____

Protein: _____

Grain: _____

THE ACTIVE CALORIE DIET JOURNAL

CARDIO WORKOUT

ACTIVITY	DURATION	INTENSITY	LOCATION

STRENGTH TRAINING

EXERCISE	WEIGHTS	REPS	COMMENTS

Active Life Habits: _____

_____

_____

_____

Active Eating Habits: _____

_____

_____

_____

Time spent sitting: _____

Food reflections: *Use this space to record what went well (and perhaps not so well) for you today.*

_____

_____

_____

My Week at a Glance

Starting weight: _____

Ending weight: _____

Total weight loss: _____

ACTIVE CALORIE SUMMARY

Total number of restaurant meals: _____

Total number of take-out meals: _____

Total number of ready-to-eat meals: _____

Total number of trips to the grocery store: _____

I tried these Active Eating Habits: _____

_____

I tried these Active Calorie foods: _____

_____

I had these Couch Potato Calorie foods: _____

_____

Thinking about the week ahead, I think my biggest challenge will be: _____

_____

ACTIVE LIFE SUMMARY

Total time I spent exercising: _____

My overall energy level for the week (circle one):   1   2   3   4   5

Total time I spent sitting this week: _____

I tried these Active Life Habits: _____

_____

_____

My favorite activity is: _____

What I learned about myself: _____

_____

_____

_____

Appendix B

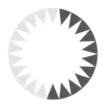

The Active Calorie Diet Sample Menus

Okay, so you're ready to chew on all this. To get you started with some tasty bites, we have included a 4-week meal plan to show you how all of this information comes together. You will see options for breakfasts, lunches, dinners, and snacks that fall within the calorie and plate balance we would like you to achieve. Each week has its own shopping checklist, so no more "sorry, don't have it, let's order a pizza" excuses!

We have also done a little mixing and matching. You'll see that some of the meal choices are from the tasty recipes in Chapter 7, some are items you may already have on hand at home, and some are good selections when you dine out. As you've learned throughout the book, this plan is designed for maximum flexibility, so feel free to adapt these meal plans to your needs, lifestyle, and tastes. If you're a vegetarian, simply swap the meat-based dishes for similar plant-based options. If you travel frequently, look for restaurant choices as well as make-ahead options that you can tote with you.

You'll see that the menus don't always match up exactly to the Active Calorie Plate guidelines. Some days you may see more than 1,500 calories, some days less; some meals have a little more protein, some a little more grain, some a little less fruits and vegetables; and so on. (And men, don't forget to add calories as needed.) Remember that the Active Calorie Plate guidelines are just that—guidelines to help you make the most active choices, not hard-and-fast rules.

That being said, here are a few more guidelines to keep in mind with these menus:

1. You can mix and match within meals, i.e., if you want waffles on Day 2 instead of Day 5, go right ahead. Feel free to swap a breakfast for a breakfast; but if a lunch choice is more appealing to you in the morning, then have a breakfast choice at lunch so you can stay within the general calorie guidelines.

2. Take a look at the preparation time for the recipes so you can plan accordingly.

3. Calories come from foods, not beverages. You'll see that most of the beverages listed in the meal plan are calorie-free (coffee, tea, sparkling water) with the exception of skim milk. If you want a soda, juice, or alcoholic beverage, you'll need to give up something else.

4. Look closely at the serving size and yield for the recipes so you eat within the appropriate calorie guidelines. If the recipe says the yield is 4 servings, and each serving equals 1 cup, then eat only 1 cup and freeze the rest or incorporate it into subsequent days. Alternatively, you can adjust the recipes to make just the number of servings you want. The shopping checklists we've provided assume that you will be making each recipe as it is written (for example, if the recipe makes 4 servings, we've listed the amounts you'll need to make 4 servings). If you choose to

adjust the recipes to make just 1 or 2 servings, be sure to adjust your shopping list amounts accordingly.

5. Although we think all the recipes are fabulous and encourage you to try each and every one, we know you're going to have favorites. If you really love the Raspberry-Almond Breakfast Parfait (page 110) and decide that is what you want every morning, like some of our participants, go for it. But try to add more variety at other meals and snacks. This will help you get all the vitamins and minerals you need. Plus, you may just discover some new favorite Active Calorie foods.

6. I know it looks like you are buying a lot, but in order to reduce waste, the shopping lists include the smallest package size for what you will need for the week. In some cases, you will have leftover ingredients. Condiments such as oils, vinegars, spices, and dried herbs will keep at least a year. Try to keep them away from heat and light to maintain freshness. Nuts, ground flaxseed, and flour can be frozen for up to a year. Bread, English muffins, tortillas, and pitas should also be frozen and can be kept for up to 6 months. Make sure the packages are tightly sealed, or transfer them to airtight containers to keep them fresher for longer and to prevent freezer burn. If you have these Active Calorie staples stocked in your kitchen, you will be encouraged and motivated to cook more regularly.

7. Most of all, ENJOY!

Active Calorie Meal Plan Week 1

Shopping List

Before you head to the grocery store, use the following checklist to see what you need to buy. You may already have many of these items on hand.

ACTIVE CALORIE PROTEINS

Ground turkey, $^1/_2$ pound

Chicken breasts, bone-in, 1 pound

Chicken breasts, skinless, boneless, $3^1/_2$ pounds

Beef fillet, 6 ounces

Ground sirloin, $^1/_2$ pound

Tilapia, halibut, or orange roughy, 6 ounces

Eggs, large, 1 dozen

Ham (from the deli counter), 2 slices, or veggie sausage

patties (such as Morningstar Farms or Boca), 1 package with 4 patties

Tuna, packed in olive oil, 3-ounce can

Salmon, 3-ounce can

ACTIVE CALORIE DAIRY

Skim milk or light soy milk, 1 quart

Nonfat Greek yogurt, plain, 1 quart

Reduced-fat sour cream, 8-ounce container

Crumbled feta, 4-ounce package

Mini Babybel Light cheese, 6-count bag

Part-skim ricotta cheese, 12 ounces

Parmesan cheese, 8 ounces

Reduced-fat Cheddar cheese, shredded, 8-ounce bag

Reduced-fat mozzarella cheese, shredded, 8-ounce bag

Low-fat Swiss cheese (from the deli counter), 1 slice

Low-fat pepper Jack or mozzarella (from the deli counter), 4 slices

ACTIVE CALORIE FRUITS

Banana, 2 small

Granny Smith apple, 1 medium

MacIntosh apple, 2 small

Mango, 1 small

Pineapple, fresh, 8-ounce container

Orange, 1 medium

Lime, 2 small

Frozen raspberries, unsweetened, 10-ounce bag

Dried cranberries, 8-ounce bag

Apple juice, 8-ounce bottle

ACTIVE CALORIE VEGETABLES

Baby spinach, 9-ounce bag

Collard greens, 1 pound

Kale, $^1/_2$ pound

Grape tomatoes, 1 pint

Red bell pepper, 2 small

Green bell pepper, 2 medium

Carrots, 1 pound (about 8 carrots)

Celery, 1 bunch (about 9 stalks)

Green beans, $1^1/_2$ pounds

Zucchini, 1 small

Broccoli, 1 large head

Bag of mixed cauliflower, broccoli, baby carrots, 16-ounce bag

Shiitake mushrooms, $^1/_2$ pound

Button mushrooms, fresh, 8-ounce container

Red onion, 1 small

Onion, 1 small

White potatoes, $1^1/_2$ pounds

Red potatoes, 2 small

Sweet potatoes, 5 medium

Cilantro, small bunch

ACTIVE CALORIE VEGETABLES (CONT.)

Parsley, small bunch

Frozen edamame, 16-ounce bag

Spicy diced tomatoes,
    15-ounce can

Cannellini beans, 8-ounce can

Kidney beans or chickpeas,
    15-ounce can

Black beans, no-salt-added,
    2 (15-ounce) cans

Marinara sauce, 12-ounce jar

ACTIVE CALORIE GRAINS

Kashi GOLEAN cereal,
    14-ounce box

Oatmeal, unflavored, 18-ounce
    canister

Popcorn, plain, microwaveable,
    or kernels, 16-ounce bag
    or jar

All Bran crackers, 10-ounce box

Brown rice, 1-pound bag or box

Whole grain or whole wheat ziti
    or penne, 2 (12-ounce) boxes

Whole grain high-fiber wraps
    (10" diameter), 6-count
    package

Whole wheat pitas (6" diameter),
    5-count package

Whole wheat baguette
    (6" long), 1

Whole wheat bread crumbs,
    12-ounce canister

Whole wheat hamburger buns,
    8-count package

Frozen whole grain waffles
    (4" square or 3" diameter),
    10-count package

ACTIVE CALORIE FATS

Walnuts, 8-ounce bag (keep in
    freezer)

Almonds, 2.25-ounce bag (keep
    in freezer)

Sesame seeds, 1-ounce bottle

Flaxseed, milled or ground,
    16-ounce box or 12-ounce
    bag (keep in freezer)

Peanut butter, chunky or
    smooth, 12-ounce jar

Bittersweet chocolate chips,
    12-ounce bag (keep in
    freezer)

Semisweet chocolate chips,
    12-ounce bag (keep in
    freezer)

Olive oil, 17-fluid-ounce bottle

Sesame seed oil, 5-ounce bottle

Light mayonnaise, 8-ounce jar

ACTIVE CALORIE ENERGIZING AND WARMING FOODS

Gingerroot, 1

Garlic bulbs, 2

Chipotle chile, 1

Jalapeño chile pepper, 1

Black pepper

Cajun seasoning

Cayenne

Chili powder

Cumin

Garlic powder

Lemon pepper

Red-pepper flakes

Balsamic vinegar

White balsamic vinegar

Adobo sauce

Spicy salsa, 16-ounce jar

Green tea

Jasmine tea

CONDIMENTS AND SEASONINGS

Cinnamon

Oregano, dried

Rosemary leaves, dried

Salt

Brown sugar

Cornstarch

Vanilla extract

Almond extract

Honey

Reduced-sodium soy sauce

Knorr's vegetable soup mix

Raspberry jam

Apple butter

Thin chocolate wafers, 9-ounce
    box (keep in freezer)

Low-sodium chicken broth,
    48-ounce box, or low-sodium
    bouillon cubes, 3.75-ounce jar

Low-sodium beef bouillon
    cubes, 14-ounce can or
    3.75-ounce jar

Red wine, 12.5-fluid-ounce
    half-bottle

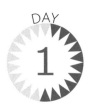

DAY 1

BREAKFAST

Peanut Butter Smoothie (page 107)

Energizing Food: Have with green tea or coffee.

LUNCH

Tuna salad: Mix together 3-ounce can of tuna in olive oil, drained; ½ cup grape tomatoes, sliced; 2 tablespoons crumbled feta cheese; and 1 tablespoon white balsamic vinegar.

18 All Bran crackers

1 small orange

Warming Food: Add some chopped hot peppers to the salad.

DINNER

Baked Ziti (page 154)

Warming Food: Add crushed red-pepper flakes to the sauce.

SNACK

2 Mini Babybel Light cheeses

1 medium Granny Smith apple

Energizing Food: Have with green tea.

DAILY TOTAL: 1,511 calories, 166 g carbs, 102 g protein, 40 g fat, 27 g fiber

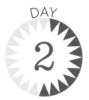

DAY

2

BREAKFAST

Apple butter waffles: Thaw 2 frozen whole wheat waffles. Top each with ½ tablespoon apple butter.

1 slice of ham or ½ veggie sausage patty

1 small apple

Energizing Food: Have with coffee or tea.

LUNCH

Chili-Topped Sweet Potato (page 145)

Warming Foods: The garlic, cumin, chipotle chile, chili powder, and adobo sauce all add heat.

DINNER

Honey-Glazed Pork Loin with Garlic Mashed Potatoes (page 169)

Warming Food: Add a dash of cayenne.

SNACK

Veggies and dip: Mix together 6 ounces plain Greek yogurt with ¼ cup crumbled feta and ¼ packet Knorr's vegetable soup mix. Serve with 2 cups of mixed vegetables, such as broccoli, cauliflower, and baby carrots.

DAILY TOTAL: 1,490 calories, 180 g carbs, 109 g protein, 40 g fat, 22 g fiber

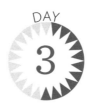

DAY

3

BREAKFAST

McDonald's Egg McMuffin

1 small banana

Energizing Food: Have with coffee or green tea.

LUNCH

Spinach salad: Mix together 3 cups spinach; 3-ounce can salmon, drained; 2 tablespoons almonds; 2 tablespoons balsamic vinegar; and ½ cup mango.

18 All Bran crackers

Warming Food: Add a dash of hot sauce.

DINNER

Fish with spicy tomatoes and onions: Top 5 ounces of halibut, tilapia, or orange roughy with ½ cup canned spicy diced tomatoes and 1 small onion, sliced. Bake at 350°F until fish is flaky, about 20 minutes. Serve with 1 cup green beans, steamed; and ½ cup brown rice cooked in low-salt chicken broth with 2 tablespoons dried cranberries added and cinnamon or powdered ginger to taste.

Warming Foods: The cinnamon or ginger adds heat.

SNACK

3 cups popcorn

2 Mini Babybel Light cheese wedges

DAILY TOTAL: 1,530 calories, 162 g carbs, 109 g protein, 35 g fat, 31 g fiber

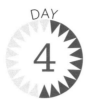

DAY

4

BREAKFAST

Southwestern Breakfast Burrito (page 115)

Warming Foods: The jalapeño and salsa in the burrito
add heat.

LUNCH

Wendy's Apple Pecan Chicken Salad

Warming Food: Add vinegar to the salad.

DINNER

Pineapple-Chicken Rice Bowl (page 156)

Warming Foods: The ginger and garlic in the rice bowl
add heat.

SNACK

SoyJoy bar

8 ounces plain nonfat Greek yogurt, flavored with
1 teaspoon almond or vanilla extract and 2 teaspoons honey

DAILY TOTAL: 1,526 calories, 167 g carbs, 113 g protein, 43 g fat, 27 g fiber

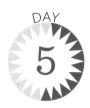

BREAKFAST

Raspberry-Almond Breakfast Parfait (page 110)

Warming Foods: The cinnamon and cayenne in the parfait add heat.

LUNCH

Six-Inch Lunch Sub (page 134)

Warming Food: The balsamic vinegar and black pepper add heat.

DINNER

Beef filet and vegetables: Broil 8-ounce beef filet to desired degree of doneness. In a nonstick skillet, sauté 1 cup each mixed broccoli, cauliflower, and carrots in 1 tablespoon olive oil. Sprinkle with red-pepper flakes to taste. Boil 2 small red potatoes and sprinkle with Cajun seasoning to taste.

Warming Food: The red-pepper flakes and Cajun seasoning add heat.

SNACK

2 Easy Ice Cream Sandwiches (page 191)

DAILY TOTAL: 1,522 calories, 182 g carbs, 97 g protein, 50 g fat, 30 g fiber

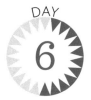

DAY

6

BREAKFAST

Oatmeal: Make ⅔ cup oatmeal, dry, with 8 ounces skim milk. Top with cinnamon to taste; ½ cup frozen berries, thawed; and 2 tablespoons walnuts.

Energizing Food: Have with coffee or green tea.

LUNCH

Chicken Minestrone (page 124)

Warming Food: The garlic adds heat, but you can also add a dash of cayenne or ginger.

DINNER

Applebee's Shrimp and Island Rice

Seasonal vegetables

Energizing Food: Have with green tea or coffee.

SNACK

Black Bean Hummus with Toasted Pita (page 180)

Warming Food: The garlic adds heat, but you can also add a dash of cayenne to the hummus.

DAILY TOTAL: 1,460 calories, 205 g carbs, 88 g protein, 32 g fat, 34 g fiber

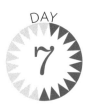

DAY

7

BREAKFAST

1 cup Kashi GOLEAN cereal with 4 ounces skim milk

1 small apple, spread with 1 tablespoon peanut butter

Energizing Food: Have with coffee or green tea.

LUNCH

Black Bean Burger (page 139)

Warming Foods: The garlic and jalapeño add heat.

DINNER

Cajun chicken: Sprinkle 6-ounce boneless, skinless chicken breast with 1 teaspoon Cajun seasoning. Spread 1 cup each chopped zucchini, mushrooms, and peppers in a single layer on a cookie sheet coated with nonstick vegetable spray. Drizzle with 1 tablespoon olive oil and ½ tablespoon balsamic vinegar. Sprinkle on red-pepper flakes and bake at 450°F for 10 minutes. Serve with ½ cup brown rice.

Warming Foods: The Cajun seasoning, crushed red-pepper flakes, and balsamic vinegar add heat.

SNACK

Sweet Potato Chips (page 181)

Warming Foods: The cayenne, garlic powder, lemon pepper, and chili powder in these chips add heat.

DAILY TOTAL: 1,484 calories, 197 g carbs, 86 g protein, 43 g fat, 34 g fiber

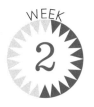

Active Calorie Meal Plan Week 2

Shopping List

Before you head to the grocery store, use the following checklist to see what you need to buy. You may already have many of these items on hand.

ACTIVE CALORIE PROTEIN

Salsa- or buffalo-flavored turkey breast, shaved or sliced (from the deli counter), 3 ounces

Turkey pepperoni (from the deli counter), $1^1/_2$ ounces

Chicken breasts, boneless, skinless, $2^1/_2$ pounds

Ham, 2 ounces

Lean beef stew meat, 1 pound

Flank steak, 6 ounces raw

Extra-lean ground beef, 8 ounces

Tilapia, 12 ounces

Shrimp, frozen or fresh, 3 pounds

Smoked salmon, 4 ounces

Eggs, large, 2 dozen

ACTIVE CALORIE DAIRY

Skim milk, 1 quart

Nonfat Greek yogurt, plain, or nonfat soy yogurt, plain, 1 quart

Nonfat Greek yogurt, fruit-flavored, 6 ounces

Part-skim mozzarella cheese, shredded, 8-ounce bag

Reduced-fat Cheddar cheese, shredded, 8-ounce bag

Laughing Cow Queso Fresco/ Chipotle cheese wedges, 1 package with 8 wedges

Crumbled feta cheese, 4-ounce container

Fat-free coffee frozen yogurt, 16-ounce container

ACTIVE CALORIE FRUITS

Bananas, 4 medium

Rome, Jonagold, or MacIntosh apples, 5 small

Red grapes, $1/_2$ pound

Pink grapefruit, 2 large

Lime, 1 small

Lemon, 1 small

Frozen sliced strawberries, unsweetened, 10-ounce bag

Frozen blueberries, unsweetened, 10-ounce bag

Dried cherries, $1/_4$ cup

Orange juice, 16-ounce bottle or carton

ACTIVE CALORIE VEGETABLES

Baby spinach, 9-ounce bag

Mixed salad greens, 10-ounce bag

Romaine lettuce, 1 large head (about 10–12 leaves)

Carrots, 1 bunch (about 8 carrots)

Celery, 1 bunch (about 9 stalks)

Tomatoes, 4 medium

Cherry tomatoes, 1 pint

Broccoli, 1 large head

Zucchini, $1/_2$ pound

Cucumber, 1 small

Red bell pepper, 1 small

Green bell pepper, 1 small

Asparagus, 1 pound

Mixed broccoli, cauliflower, and carrots, 12-ounce bag

Hass avocados, 2

Button mushrooms, fresh, 8 ounces

Shallots, 3

Yellow onion, 2 small

White potatoes, 3 medium

Fresh basil, small bunch

Fresh dill, small bunch

Fresh parsley, small bunch

Frozen peas, 2 (10-ounce) bags

Frozen artichokes, 8-ounce
package

Frozen sweet potato fries,
1 pound

Diced tomatoes, 15-ounce can

Chopped tomatoes, no-salt-
added, 15-ounce can

Tomato paste, 4-ounce can

Black beans, no-salt-added,
15-ounce can

ACTIVE CALORIE GRAINS

Oatmeal, regular, 18-ounce
container

Bran flakes, 16-ounce box

Fresh whole wheat linguine,
$1/2$ pound

Raw soba noodles, 12 ounces

Whole wheat bread, sliced, 1 bag
(keep in freezer)

Mini whole grain rolls
($2^1/_2$" diameter), 2

Whole wheat pitas
(6" diameter), 2 (5-count)
bags (keep in freezer)

Whole grain tortillas
(6" diameter), 2 (12-count)
packages

Short-grain brown rice, 1-pound
box or bag

Buckwheat pancake mix,
32-ounce box

Yellow cake mix, 10.25-ounce
box

Whole wheat flour, 5-pound bag
(keep in freezer)

Frozen whole wheat pizza
dough, 1 pound

ACTIVE CALORIE FATS

Reduced-fat coconut milk,
16-ounce can

Chopped pecans, 2-ounce bag
(keep in freezer)

Almond butter, 12-ounce jar

Peanut butter, 12-ounce jar

Ground flaxseed, 12-ounce box
or bag (keep in freezer)

Sesame seeds, 1 ounce

Canola oil, 16-ounce bottle

Olive oil, 16 ounces

Sesame seed oil, 5 ounces

Light mayonnaise, 8-ounce jar

Unsalted butter, 2 sticks

ACTIVE CALORIE ENERGIZING AND WARMING FOODS

Gingerroot, 1

Jalapeño chile pepper or
Holland pepper, 1

Garlic bulb, 1

Pickled jalapeño chile peppers,
12 ounces

Black pepper

Cayenne

Chili powder

Cinnamon

Hot sauce

Spicy salsa, 16-ounce jar

Spicy BBQ sauce, 16-ounce jar

Apple cider vinegar, 16-ounce
bottle

Malt vinegar, 12-ounce bottle

Dijon mustard, 7.5 ounces

ACTIVE CALORIE CONDIMENTS

Allspice

Dried onions

Oregano

Paprika

Pumpkin pie spice

Salt

Baking powder

Baking soda

Cornstarch

Sugar, 16-ounce bag or box

Light brown sugar, 16-ounce
bag or box

Honey

Maple syrup

Molasses

Fat-free caramel sauce, 8 ounces

Raspberry jam

Strawberry Simply Fruit spread,
10-ounce jar

Vanilla extract

Sweet pickle relish, 10-ounce jar

Lemon juice

Low-sodium soy sauce,
10 ounces

Reduced-sodium beef broth,
24-ounce carton

White wine, 12.5 fl oz

Amaretto or other almond-
flavored liqueur, 1 fluid ounce

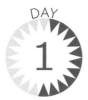

DAY

1

BREAKFAST

Cookie-Crunch Smoothie (page 106)

Energizing and Warming Foods: Have with coffee or tea. Add cinnamon to the smoothie.

LUNCH

Spicy turkey wrap: Spread 1 Laughing Cow Light Spicy Queso Fresco/Chipolte cheese wedge on a 6" whole wheat tortilla. Top with 3 ounces salsa deli turkey breast, shaved or sliced, and ½ cup baby spinach leaves. Roll up and eat. Have with 1½ cups red grapes.

Warming Food: The spice in the turkey breast adds heat.

DINNER

Peanut Noodles (page 175)

Warming Foods: The garlic and hot sauce in the noodles add heat.

SNACK

Raspberry-Filled Oat Bar (page 183)

Energizing and Warming Foods: Have with green tea. The cinnamon and cayenne in the bar add heat.

DAILY TOTAL: 1,547 calories, 235 g carbs, 74 g protein, 36 g fat, 19 g fiber

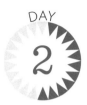

DAY

2

BREAKFAST

Cinnamon-ginger oatmeal: Make ½ cup oatmeal with
8 ounces skim milk. Add 1 teaspoon grated fresh ginger,
½ teaspoon cinnamon, and cook. Mix in 1 small chopped
apple, 1 tablespoon pecans, and 1 teaspoon maple syrup.

Energizing and Warming Foods: Have with coffee or tea.
The ginger and cinnamon in the oatmeal add heat.

LUNCH

Pizzette with Arrabiata Sauce (page 143)

Warming Foods: The jalapeño and garlic in the sauce add
heat.

DINNER

Orange-Sesame Chicken (page 164)

Warming Foods: The vinegar, garlic, ginger, and red-pepper
flakes add heat.

SNACK

6 ounces fruit-flavored Greek or low-fat soy yogurt, topped
with 2 tablespoons bran flakes and ½ cup unsweetened
blueberries, fresh or frozen.

DAILY TOTAL: 1,492 calories, 228 g carbs, 75 g protein, 33 g fat, 36 g fiber

DAY

3

BREAKFAST

Ham-and-Cheese Bake (page 116)

Warming Food: Add hot sauce to taste.

LUNCH

Avocado Seafood Salad (page 132)

Warming Foods: The cayenne, black pepper, and mustard add heat.

DINNER

Hungarian Beef Stew (page 167)

Warming Food: The hot paprika or cayenne adds heat.

SNACK

2 cups Almond Butter Caramel Corn (page 187)

DAILY TOTAL: 1,468 calories, 162 g carbs, 102 g protein, 45 g fat, 25 g fiber

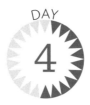

BREAKFAST

2 Zucchini-Apple Muffins (page 121)

Energizing and Warming Foods: The cinnamon in the muffins adds heat. Have with coffee or green tea.

LUNCH

Egg Salad (page 127)

Warming Food: Add a dash of cayenne or hot sauce to the egg salad.

DINNER

Flank steak fajitas: Grill or broil 4 ounces flank steak. In nonstick skillet with 1 tablespoon olive oil, sauté ½ cup each thinly sliced onions and mushrooms, and red and green peppers until tender. Place thinly sliced steak and vegetables into a 6"-diameter whole wheat tortilla and top with ¼ cup spicy salsa.

Warming Food: The spicy salsa gives this some heat.

SNACK

Coffee Bananas Foster (page 185)

Warming Foods: The cinnamon and cayenne add heat.

DAILY TOTAL: 1,509 calories, 212 g carbs, 67 g protein, 42 g fat, 24 g fiber

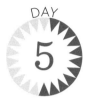

DAY

5

BREAKFAST

Waffles with strawberries: Mix ⅓ cup part-skim ricotta with 1 tablespoon Strawberry Simply Fruit spread. Top 2 whole grain waffles with ricotta mixture and ½ cup sliced strawberries.

Energizing Food: Have with coffee or tea.

LUNCH

Wendy's Grilled Chicken Sandwich

Wendy's Side Salad with 1 packet fat-free French dressing

Warming Food: Add hot sauce to the chicken sandwich.

DINNER

Fish and Chips (page 170)

Warming Food: The vinegar adds heat.

SNACK

Black Bean Hummus with Toasted Pita (page 180)

Warming Food: The garlic adds heat, but you can also add a dash of cayenne to the hummus.

DAILY TOTAL: 1,482 calories, 196 g carbs, 80 g protein, 45 g fat, 21 g fiber

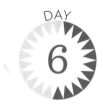

DAY

6

BREAKFAST

Buckwheat Pancakes with Smoked Salmon (page 118)

Warming Food: The cayenne adds heat.

LUNCH

Spicy Chicken Tacos (page 135)

Warming Foods: The garlic, cumin, chili powder, cayenne, and jalapeños add heat.

DINNER

Sliders: Divide 6 ounces raw, extra-lean ground beef into 2 small patties. Broil until done. Cut 2 mini whole wheat rolls (2½"-diameter) in half. On each roll, place 1 hamburger patty; ⅛ avocado; ½ small onion, sliced; and 1 tablespoon spicy barbecue sauce.

½ cup each broccoli, cauliflower, and carrots, steamed.

Warming Food: The spice in the barbecue sauce adds heat.

SNACK

Caramel Apple Cake (page 184)

Warming Foods: The cinnamon, cayenne, and ginger add heat.

DAILY TOTAL: 1,537 calories, 173 g carbs, 112 g protein, 38 g fat, 42 g fiber

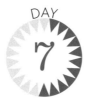

DAY

7

BREAKFAST

1 medium banana spread with 2 tablespoons creamy or chunky peanut butter

6 ounces fruit-flavored Greek yogurt

Energizing Food: Have with coffee or tea.

LUNCH

Pepperoni Calzone (page 141)

Warming Food: Add a dash of hot sauce or crushed red-pepper flakes.

DINNER

Shrimp Scampi Linguine (page 174)

Warming Foods: The garlic and red-pepper flakes add heat.

SNACK

½ whole wheat pita spread with 2 Laughing Cow Queso Fresco/Chipotle cheese wedges.

DAILY TOTAL: 1,472 calories, 184 g carbs, 91 g protein, 43 g fat, 29 g fiber

WEEK

3 Active Calories Meal Plan Week 3

Shopping List

Before you head to the grocery store, use the following checklist to see what you need to buy. You may already have many of these items on hand.

ACTIVE CALORIE PROTEIN

Chicken cutlets, boneless, skinless, 1 pound

Chicken breasts, boneless, skinless, 3 pounds

Ground turkey breast, 12 ounces

Flank steak, 10 ounces raw weight

Tri tip or eye of round (cut into 6 cubes), 6 ounces raw weight

Baked ham, 2 slices

Turkey bacon, nitrate-free, 12-ounce package

Cod fillets, boneless, 1 pound

Shrimp, medium, $^1/_2$ pound

Eggs, large, 2 dozen

Tuna, packed in olive oil, 3-ounce can

BiPro Whey Protein Isolate, unflavored, 1 (22-gram) packet

ACTIVE CALORIE DAIRY

Skim milk, 1 quart + 12 ounces, or $^1/_2$ gallon

Nonfat Greek yogurt, plain, 8 ounces

Low-fat sour cream, 8 ounces

1% cottage cheese, 4 ounces

Part-skim ricotta cheese, 12-ounce container

Parmesan cheese, grated, 12 ounces

Mozzarella cheese, shredded, 8-ounce bag

Low-fat Cheddar cheese, shredded, 12-ounce bag

Feta cheese, crumbled, 4 ounces

Boccoccini (mini fresh mozzarella balls), 12-ounce container

ACTIVE CALORIE FRUITS

Banana, 1 small

Granny Smith apple, 1 small

MacIntosh apple, 2 small

Blueberries, 1 pint

Strawberries, 3 large

Raspberries, $^1/_2$ pint

Oranges, 2 large + 1 small

Lemon, 2 small

Frozen blueberries, 10-ounce bag

ACTIVE CALORIE VEGETABLES

Baby spinach, 9-ounce bag

Romaine lettuce, 4 large heads

Radicchio, 10-ounce head

French green beans, $^1/_2$ pound

Green bell pepper, 2 medium

Red bell pepper, 2 medium

Asparagus, $3^1/_2$ pounds

Brussels sprouts, $^1/_2$ pound

Broccoli, 2 medium heads

Zucchini, 1 medium

Carrots, 1 bunch (about 8 carrots)

Celery, 1 bunch (about 9 stalks)

Tomatoes, 10 medium

Plum tomatoes, 4 medium

Cherry tomatoes, 1 pint

Hass avocado, 1 ripe

Button mushrooms, 8

Shiitake mushrooms, 6 ounces

Scallions, 4 stalks

Yellow onion, 1 medium

Red onions, 3 medium

Red potatoes, 2 small

Russet potatoes, 2 pounds

Idaho potatoes, 4 (2 pounds)

Sweet potato, 1 medium

Fresh basil, small bunch

ACTIVE CALORIE VEGETABLES (CONT.)

Fresh parsley, small bunch

Fresh rosemary, small bunch

Fresh thyme leaves, small bunch

Roasted red peppers,
12-ounce jar

Frozen artichokes, 8-ounce
package

Lentils, green or French,
16-ounce bag

Garbanzo beans, 8-ounce can

Marinara sauce, 12-ounce jar

Guiltless Gourmet or Desert
Pepper black bean dip,
16-ounce jar

ACTIVE CALORIE GRAINS

Wheatena cereal, 20-ounce box

Fresh whole wheat pasta,
8-ounce package

Whole grain or brown rice pasta,
12-ounce box

Soba noodles, 8 ounces

Whole grain English muffins,
6 (keep in freezer)

Country-style whole wheat
bread, high-fiber, 1 loaf (keep
in freezer)

Whole wheat baguette
(6" long), 1

Whole wheat tortillas
(8" diameter), 1 package with
10 tortillas (keep in freezer)

Short-grain brown rice, 16-ounce
bag or box

Whole wheat flour, 5-pound bag
(keep in freezer)

Whole wheat bread crumbs,
12-ounce container

Corn muffin mix, 8.5-ounce box

Baked tortilla chips, 1-ounce bag

Thin chocolate wafers, 9-ounce
box (keep in freezer)

ACTIVE CALORIE FATS

Green olives, 5.75 ounces

Cashew pieces, 8-ounce bag
(keep in freezer)

Chopped walnuts, 2-ounce bag
(keep in freezer)

Chunky peanut butter, 12 ounces

Ground flaxseed, 12- or
16-ounce bag or box (keep in
freezer)

Semisweet chocolate pieces,
8-ounce bag (keep in freezer)

Olive oil, 17 ounces

Canola oil, 16 ounces

Unsalted butter, 1 stick ($\frac{1}{2}$ cup)

ACTIVE CALORIE ENERGIZING AND WARMING FOODS

Pappadew peppers or roasted
red peppers, 12-ounce jar

Garlic bulb, 1

Jalapeño peppers, 2

Chipotle chili in adobo sauce

Black pepper

Cayenne pepper

Cinnamon

Chili powder

Crushed red-pepper flakes

Garlic powder

Powdered ginger

Hot sauce

Spicy salsa, 12-ounce jar

Dijon mustard

Apple cider vinegar, 8-ounce
bottle

Balsamic vinegar, 8-ounce bottle

Red wine vinegar, 8-ounce
bottle

Rice vinegar, 8-ounce bottle

CONDIMENTS AND SEASONINGS

Dried onions

Italian seasoning

Salt

Powdered sugar, 1 pound

Sugar

Cornstarch

Vanilla extract

Blueberry Simply Fruit spread,
12-ounce bottle

Raspberry jam

Honey

Barbecue sauce

Cocktail sauce

Oyster sauce, 9-ounce bottle

Worcestershire sauce

Reduced-sodium chicken broth,
15-ounce can

White wine, 12.5 fluid ounces

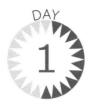

DAY
1

BREAKFAST

Strawberries-and-Cream Hot Cereal (page 109)

Energizing Food: Have with coffee or tea.

LUNCH

Salad niçoise: Top 1 cup French green beans, steamed, 1 hard-cooked egg, chopped, and 2 small red potatoes, boiled and cut into quarters, with 3-ounce can tuna in olive oil, drained. Dress with 1 tablespoon balsamic vinegar. Serve with small Granny Smith apple.

Warming Food: The vinegar adds some heat. You can also add a dash of hot sauce to the salad.

DINNER

Bacon-and-Broccoli Bow Ties (page 159)

Warming Foods: The vinegar and garlic add heat.

SNACK

Corn Muffin with Colby and Jalapeño (page 182)

Warming Food: The jalapeño adds heat.

DAILY TOTAL: 1,535 calories, 202 g carbs, 86 g protein, 41 g fat, 34 g fiber

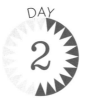

DAY

2

BREAKFAST

Eggs and Tomatoes (page 112)

Warming Food: The red-pepper flakes add heat.

LUNCH

Steak Burrito (page 136)

Warming Foods: The chipotle chile, adobo sauce, garlic, and spicy salsa add heat.

DINNER

Cashew Chicken (page 165)

Energizing and Warming Food: Have with green tea. The vinegar and garlic add heat.

SNACK

Chips and dip: Mix ¼ cup black bean dip (spicy Guiltless Gourmet or Desert Pepper) with ½ cup spicy salsa. Enjoy with 12 baked tortilla chips.

Warming Food: The spices in the salsa add heat.

DAILY TOTAL: 1,468 calories, 189 g carbs, 82 g protein, 40 g fat, 31 g fiber

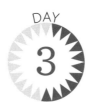
DAY

3

BREAKFAST

Bacon-and-Broccoli Egg Sandwich (page 113)

Warming Food: The hot sauce adds heat.

LUNCH

California Salad (page 128)

Warming Foods: The chili powder, garlic powder, black pepper, vinegar, and mustard all add heat.

DINNER

Shepherd's Pie (page 161)

Warming Food: The chili powder adds heat.

SNACK

2 Easy Ice Cream Sandwiches (page 191)

DAILY TOTAL: 1,542 calories, 203 g carbs, 93 g protein, 34 g fat, 31 g fiber

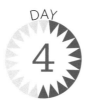

DAY

4

BREAKFAST

Stuffed Blueberry French Toast (page 117)

Energizing Food: Have with coffee or green tea.

LUNCH

Twice-Cooked Potato Skins (page 144)

Warming Foods: The hot sauce and garlic powder add heat.

DINNER

Balsamic Chicken and Pasta (page 160)

Warming Foods: The black pepper, red-pepper flakes, and balsamic vinegar add heat.

SNACK

Corn Muffin with Colby and Jalapeño (page 182)

Warming Food: The jalapeño adds heat.

DAILY TOTAL: 1,499 calories, 171 g carbs, 90 g protein, 35 g fat, 27 g fiber

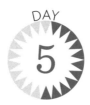

BREAKFAST

Coffee smoothie: Blend 8 ounces coffee, 4 ounces skim milk, 1 teaspoon sugar, crushed ice, and cinnamon to taste.

Blueberry Wheatena: Cook 3 tablespoons Wheatena according to package directions. Add ½ cup blueberries, 1 tablespoon Blueberry Simply Fruit spread, 1 tablespoon chopped cashews, and cinnamon to taste.

Energizing and Warming Foods: The coffee is energizing. The cinnamon adds heat.

LUNCH

Qdoba vegetarian tortilla soup (ask for no sour cream)

Qdoba soft shredded beef taco (ask for extra beef, grilled, and fajita vegetables, lettuce, black beans, pico de gallo, fiery habanero sauce)

Warming Food: The fiery habanero sauce adds heat.

DINNER

Fish in a Packet with Hot Buttered Rice (page 171)

Warming Foods: The garlic and Peppadew peppers add heat.

SNACK

2 Easy Ice Cream Sandwiches (page 191)

DAILY TOTAL: 1,471 calories, 206 g carbs, 70 g protein, 39 g fat, 24 g fiber

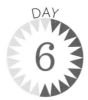
DAY

6

BREAKFAST

Ricotta-berry toast: In a small bowl, mix ½ cup part-skim ricotta, 1 teaspoon vanilla extract, 1 tablespoon Blueberry Simply Fruit spread, ½ cup frozen or fresh blueberries, and ginger to taste. Spread on 2 slices of whole wheat toast.

Energizing and Warming Foods: Have coffee or green tea. The ginger adds heat.

LUNCH

Shrimp Cocktail on Toast (page 142)

Warming Food: The garlic gives some heat, but add a dash of hot sauce or wasabi for even more.

DINNER

Beef kebabs: Cut 4 ounces tri tip or eye of round beef into 6 cubes. Prepare 2 skewers, each with 2 chunks of zucchini, 2 chunks of pepper, 2 pieces of meat, 1 piece of mushroom, 1 wedge of onion (in any order). Marinate in a mix of 2 tablespoons balsamic vinegar, 1 tablespoon olive oil, powdered ginger, crushed red-pepper flakes to taste. Grill or broil the kebabs. Serve over ½ cup brown rice.

Warming Foods: The vinegar, ginger, and red-pepper flakes add heat.

SNACK

1 small apple with 1 tablespoon chunky or creamy peanut butter

DAILY TOTAL: 1,476 calories, 170 g carbs, 112 g protein, 56 g fat, 24 g fiber

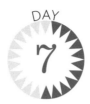

DAY

7

BREAKFAST

Ham and cheese sandwich: Top each half of a whole wheat
English muffin with 1 slice baked ham and ¼ cup shredded
light Cheddar. Broil until the cheese melts.

1 small orange

Warming Food: Have with green tea.

LUNCH

Barbecue Chicken Salad (page 131)

Warming Foods: The chipotle chile and adobo sauce add heat.

DINNER

Frittata: In a nonstick pan in 1 tablespoon olive oil, sauté until
tender ½ cup mushrooms, ½ cup red bell pepper, ¼ cup onions,
all chopped. Add ½ cup baby spinach and ½ cup garbanzo
beans. Sauté 1 minute. Remove from heat. In a separate bowl,
beat 3 eggs with 1 tablespoon water, Italian seasoning, cayenne,
salt, and black pepper to taste. Pour over the vegetables, sprinkle
1 tablespoon grated Parmesan, and cook until set. Top with
½ cup salsa and serve with a baked sweet potato.

Warming Foods: The cayenne and black pepper add heat.

SNACK

Banana shake: Blend 6 ounces skim milk; 1 small banana, frozen;
1 teaspoon vanilla extract; a dash of cinnamon; and 2 teaspoons
honey.

DAILY TOTAL: 1,521 calories, 142 g carbs, 97 g protein, 59 g fat, 26 g fiber

4   Active Calorie Meal Plan Week 4

Shopping List

Before you head to the grocery store, use the following checklist to see what you need to buy. You may already have many of these items on hand.

ACTIVE CALORIE PROTEIN

Chicken breasts, boneless, skinless, 4 pounds

Chicken thighs, boneless, skinless, 2

Chicken cutlets, thinly sliced, 1 pound

Ground turkey breast, 8 ounces

Ground turkey, 1 pound

Pork loin, 3 ounces raw

Baked ham, low-sodium, 1 ounce

Salmon fillets, 2 pounds

Eggs, large, 2 dozen

Tuna, packed in spring water, 2 (5-ounce) cans

ACTIVE CALORIE DAIRY

Skim milk, 1 quart

Nonfat Greek yogurt, plain, 1 quart

Reduced-fat sour cream, 12-ounce container

Low-fat Cheddar cheese, shredded, 16-ounce bag

Part-skim ricotta, 12-ounce container

Part-skim mozzarella cheese, shredded, 8-ounce bag

Brie, 1/4 pound

Crumbled blue cheese, 4-ounce container

Parmesan cheese, grated, 12-ounce container

ACTIVE CALORIE FRUITS

Bananas, 3 small

Apple, 1 small

Mangoes, 2 small

Strawberries, 1 pint

Blueberries, fresh, 1 pint, or frozen, 12-ounce bag

Oranges, 5 medium

Lemons, 2 small

Lime, 1 small

Dried cherries, 1/3 cup

Raisins, 12-ounce bag, 15-ounce box, or 1 package of 6 (1-ounce) boxes

ACTIVE CALORIE VEGETABLES

Baby spinach, 9-ounce bag

Romaine lettuce, 2 large heads

Red cabbage, 1 small head

Radicchio, 1-pound head

Green beans, 1 1/4 pounds

Orange bell pepper, 1 medium

Carrots, bunch (about 8 carrots)

Grape tomatoes, 1 pint

Tomatoes, 3 medium

Broccoli, 1 large head

Zucchini, 5 small

Portabello mushroom, 1 large

Red onions, 3 small

Yellow onion, 1 large

Scallions, 4 stalks

Shallot, 1 large

Sweet potatoes, 10

Fresh basil, small bunch

Fresh chives, small bunch

Fresh mint, small bunch

Fresh parsley, small bunch

Fresh tarragon or basil, small container

Fresh thyme, small container

Frozen artichokes, 8-ounce bag

Amy's Roasted Vegetable Lasagna, frozen

ACTIVE CALORIE VEGETABLES (CONT.)

Artichokes, 8-ounce can

Diced tomatoes, no-salt-added, 28-ounce can

Whole peeled tomatoes, no-salt-added, 28-ounce can

Salsa verde, 17.6-ounce jar

Black beans, no-salt-added, 15-ounce can

Cannellini beans, no-salt-added, 2 (15-ounce) cans

ACTIVE CALORIE GRAINS

Banana SOYJOY bar, 1

Kashi GOLEAN Cereal, 14-ounce box

Whole wheat bread crumbs, seasoned, 12 ounces

Whole wheat bread, high-fiber, 1 loaf (keep in freezer)

Whole wheat hoagie rolls (6" long), 4

Small whole wheat baguette (6" long), 2

Whole wheat pitas (6" diameter), 5-count package

Whole wheat tortillas (10" diameter), 10-count package

Whole wheat couscous, 11-ounce box

Whole wheat angel hair pasta, 12-ounce box

Brown rice, 1-pound box or bag

Whole wheat flour, 5-pound bag (keep in freezer)

Corn muffin mix, 8.5-ounce box

Whole wheat pancake mix, 32-ounce box

Popcorn kernels, 1-pound bag or box

Wheat Thins, 10-ounce box

Wonton wrappers, frozen, 1 pound

ACTIVE CALORIE FATS

Walnuts, 2 ounces

Pecans, chopped, 2-ounce bag

Golden flaxseed, ground, 16-ounce bag or 12-ounce box (keep in freezer)

Pine nuts, 2 ounces

Almond butter

Olive oil

Unsalted butter, 1 stick ($1/2$ cup)

Light mayonnaise, 8-ounce jar

ACTIVE CALORIE HEAT AND ENERGIZE FOODS

Poblano peppers, 4

Jalapeño chile peppers, 6

Garlic bulb, 1

Black pepper

Cayenne

Chili powder

Cinnamon

Curry powder

Garlic powder

Lemon pepper

Hot sauce

Balsamic vinegar

Wasabi peas, $1/2$ cup

CONDIMENTS AND SEASONINGS

Allspice

Ground cardamom

Paprika

Pumpkin pie spice

Baking soda

Baking powder

Salt

Sugar

Light brown sugar

Star anise pods, 2

Vanilla extract

Honey

Maple syrup

Molasses

Barbecue sauce

Sweet pickle relish

Worcestershire sauce

Reduced-sodium soy sauce

Low-sodium chicken broth, 15-ounce can

DAY

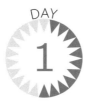

1

BREAKFAST

Birdies in a Basket (page 114)

Warming Foods: The black pepper and cayenne add heat.

LUNCH

Taco Salad (page 129)

Warming Foods: The hot sauce adds heat.

DINNER

No-Boil Manicotti (page 155)

Warming Foods: Add a dash of cayenne pepper.

SNACK

Banana SOYJOY bar

4 ounces plain nonfat Greek yogurt flavored with a splash of vanilla and 1 teaspoon honey

DAILY TOTAL: 1,546 calories, 185 g carbs, 94 g protein, 42 g fat, 35 g fiber

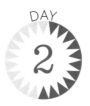

DAY

2

BREAKFAST

Blueberry-Walnut Pancakes with Cardamom (page 119)

Energizing and Warming Foods: Have with coffee or green tea. If you choose to use cinnamon instead of cardamom, it adds heat.

LUNCH

Strawberry Salmon (page 147)

Warming Foods: The black pepper, cayenne, and vinegar add heat.

DINNER

Stuffed-Pepper Bake (page 166)

Warming Foods: Add a dash of ground black pepper or cayenne.

SNACK

2 cups Almond Butter Caramel Corn (page 187)

DAILY TOTAL: 1,492 calories, 215 g carbs, 70 g protein, 48 g fat, 26 g fiber

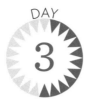

BREAKFAST

2 Zucchini-Apple Muffins (page 121)

Energizing and Warming Foods: The cinnamon in the muffins adds heat. Have with coffee or green tea.

LUNCH

Pulled BBQ Chicken Sandwich (page 138)

Warming Food: Add a dash of cayenne.

DINNER

Amy's Roasted Vegetable Lasagna frozen entrée

Cannellini bean salad: Top 1 cup Romaine lettuce with ½ cup cannellini beans, ½ cup grape tomatoes, and 1 tablespoon balsamic vinegar.

Warming Foods: The balsamic vinegar adds heat, but you can also add crushed red-pepper flakes or hot sauce to the salad or lasagna.

SNACK

Sweet Potato Chips (page 181)

Warming Food: The cayenne, lemon pepper, garlic powder, and chili powder in these chips add heat.

DAILY TOTAL: 1,492 calories, 215 g carbs, 70 g protein, 48 g fat, 26 g fiber

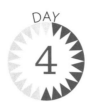

DAY

4

BREAKFAST

1 cup Kashi GOLEAN cereal

6 ounces skim milk

2 tablespoons raisins

Warming Food: Have with green tea.

LUNCH

Tropical Salad (page 133)

Warming Foods: The cumin in the curry powder and the hot sauce add heat.

DINNER

Orange-Soy Salmon (page 172)

Energizing Food: Have with green tea.

SNACK

2 cups Almond Butter Caramel Corn (page 187)

DAILY TOTAL: 1,459 calories, 224 g carbs, 70 g protein, 36 g fat, 28 g fiber

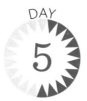

DAY

5

BREAKFAST

French Scrambled Eggs (page 111)

Warming Food: Add a dash of cayenne.

LUNCH

Tuna Salad Crunch (page 130)

Warming Foods: The black pepper, jalapeño, and wasabi peas all add heat.

DINNER

Chicken-Pesto Parmesan (page 163)

Warming Food: The garlic adds some heat, but add a dash of cayenne for more.

SNACK

Corn Muffin with Colby and Jalapeño (page 182)

Warming Food: The jalapeño in the muffin gives it heat.

DAILY TOTAL: 1,464 calories, 169 g carbs, 94 g protein, 39 g fat, 28 g fiber

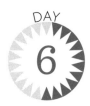

BREAKFAST

Blueberry smoothie: Blend together 8 ounces skim milk,
½ cup frozen blueberries, ½ cup plain nonfat Greek yogurt,
2 teaspoons honey, 1 teaspoon vanilla extract, and cinnamon to taste.

1 small banana with 1 tablespoon almond butter

Energizing Food: Have with coffee or green tea.

LUNCH

Subway Red Wine Vinaigrette Club (6")

Warming Food: Ask for extra jalapeño peppers.

DINNER

Moist Meat Loaf with Sweet Potato Mash (page 168)

Warming Foods: The garlic and hot sauce add heat.

SNACK

1 cup Kashi GOLEAN cereal with 6 ounces skim milk

DAILY TOTAL: 1,511 calories, 224 g carbs, 94 g protein, 31 g fat, 26 g fiber

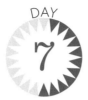

DAY

7

BREAKFAST

Spread 2 tablespoons salsa on 1 Corn Muffin with Colby and Jalapeño (page 182), split and filled with 2 scrambled eggs

1 small orange

Warming Foods: The jalapeños in the muffin add heat.

LUNCH

Cuban Sandwich (page 137)

Warming Food: Add a dash of hot sauce.

DINNER

Lemon garlic chicken: Sauté 1 clove garlic, minced, in 1 teaspoon olive oil until golden. Add 2 small chicken thighs and brown. Add juice from 1 lemon and ¼ teaspoon lemon zest, sprinkle on 1 teaspoon chopped fresh thyme, and cook until done. Add salt and black pepper to taste. Cook ¼ cup whole wheat couscous in low-salt chicken broth and add 1 tablespoon each chopped pecans and dried cherries. Serve with 1 cup steamed green beans.

Warming Food: The black pepper adds heat.

SNACK

Sweet Potato Chips (page 181)

Warming Foods: The cayenne, lemon pepper, garlic powder, and chili powder in these chips add heat.

DAILY TOTAL: 1,508 calories, 150 g carbs, 90 g protein, 44 g fat, 22 g fiber

Endnotes

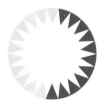

INTRODUCTION

1   G. N. Healy, MPH; D. W. Dunstan, PhD; J. Salmon, PhD; E. Cerin, PhD; J. E. Shaw, MD; P. Z. Zimmet, MD; and N. Owen, PhD, "Breaks in Sedentary Time: Beneficial Associations with Metabolic Risks," *Diabetes Care* 31, no. 4 (April 2008): 661–66.
2   P. T. Katzmarzyk, T. S. Church, C. L. Craig, and C. Bouchard, "Sitting Time and Mortality from All Causes, Cardiovascular Disease, and Cancer," *Medicine & Science in Sports & Exercise* 41, no. 5 (May 2009): 998–1005.

CHAPTER 1

1   K. Murakami, S. Sasaki, Y. Takahashi, K. Uenishi, M. Yamasaki, H. Hayabuchi, T. Goda, J. Oka, K. Baba, K. Ohki, T. Kohri, K. Muramatsu, and M. Furuki, "Hardness (Difficulty of Chewing) of the Habitual Diet in Relation to Body Mass Index and Waist Circumference in Free-Living Japanese Women Aged 18–22 Y[ears]," *American Journal of Clinical Nutrition* 86, no. 1 (July 2007): 206–13.
2   K. Oka, A. Sakuarae1, T. Fujise, H. Yoshimatsu, T. Sakata, and M. Nakata, "Food Texture Differences Affect Energy Metabolism in Rats," *Journal of Dental Research* 82, no. 6 (February 2003): 491–94.
3   E. J. Stevenson, N. M. Astbury, E. J. Simpson, M. A. Taylor, and I. A. Macdonald, "Fat Oxidation during Exercise and Satiety during Recovery Are Increased following a Low-Glycemic Index Breakfast in Sedentary Women," *Journal of Nutrition* 139, no. 5 (May 2009): 890–97.
4   C. R. Bulik, PhD, William R. and Jeanne H. Jordan Distinguished Professor of Eating Disorders in the UNC School of Medicine's department of psychiatry and director of the UNC Eating Disorders Program (presentation of survey in collaboration with *SELF*, Academy for Eating Disorders' 2008 International Conference on Eating Disorders, Seattle, May 17).
5   A. J. Smeets and M. S. Westerterp-Plantenga, "Acute Effects on Metabolism and Appetite Profile of One Meal Difference in the Lower Range of Meal Frequency," *British Journal of Nutrition* 99, no. 6 (June 2008): 1316–21.
6   L. R. Purslow, M. S. Sandhu, N. Forouhi, E. H. Young, R. N. Luben, A. A. Welch, K. Khaw, S. A. Bingham, and N. J. Wareham, "Energy Intake at Breakfast and

Weight Change: Prospective Study of 6,764 Middle-Aged Men and Women," *American Journal of Epidemiology* 167, no. 2 (January 2008): 188–92.

7   Y. Ma, E. R. Bertone, E. J. Stanek III, G. W. Reed, J. R. Hebert, N. L. Cohen, P. A. Merriam, and I. S. Ockene, "Association between Eating Patterns and Obesity in a Free-Living US Adult Population," *American Journal of Epidemiology* 158, no. 1 (July 2003): 85–92.

CHAPTER 2

1   J. Levine, MB, BS, PhD, and I. Pavlidis, PhD, "The Energy Expended in Chewing Gum," *New England Journal of Medicine* 341 (December 30, 1999): 2100.

2   See https://biolincc.nhlbi.nih.gov/studies/omniheart/

3   L. Brookes, MSc, "OmniHeart—Optimal Macronutrient Intake Trial to Prevent Heart Disease," Medscape CME © 2006 Medscape, LLC, http://cme.medscape.com/viewarticle/523041.

4   R. J. de Souza, J. F. Swain, L. J. Appel, and F. M. Sacks, "Alternatives for Macronutrient Intake and Chronic Disease: A Comparison of the OmniHeart Diets with Popular Diets and with Dietary Recommendations," *American Journal of Clinical Nutrition* 88, no. 1 (July 2008): 1–11.

5   D. S. Weigle, P. A. Breen, C. C. Matthys, H. S. Callahan, K. E. Meeuws, V. R. Burden, and J. Q. Purnell, "A High-Protein Diet Induces Sustained Reductions in Appetite, Ad Libitum Caloric Intake, and Body Weight Despite Compensatory Changes in Diurnal Plasma Leptin and Ghrelin Concentrations," *American Journal of Clinical Nutrition* 82, no. 1 (July 2005): 41–48.

6   J. S. Vander Wal, A. Gupta, P. Khosla, and N. V. Dhurandhar, "Egg Breakfast Enhances Weight Loss," *International Journal of Obesity* 32 (2008): 1545–51; published online August 5, 2008.

7   K. J. Hackney, A. J. Bruenger, and J. T. Lemmer, "Timing Protein Intake Increases Energy Expenditure 24 H[ours] after Resistance Training," *Medicine & Science in Sports & Exercise* 42, no. 5 (May 2010): 998–1003.

8   A. R. Josse, J. E. Tang, M. A. Tarnopolsky, and S. M. Phillips. "Body Composition and Strength Changes in Women with Milk and Resistance Exercise," *Medicine & Science in Sport & Exercise* 42, no. 6 (June 2010): 1122–30.

9   J. A. Higgins, D. R. Higbee, W. T. Donahoo, I. L. Brown, M. L. Bell, and D. H. Bessesen, "Resistant Starch Consumption Promotes Lipid Oxidation," *Nutrition & Metabolism* 1, no. 8 (October 2004), http://www.nutritionandmetabolism.com/content/1/1/8.

10 K. McManus, L. Antinoro, and F. Sacks, "A Randomized Controlled Trial of a Moderate-Fat, Low-Energy Diet Compared with a Low Fat, Low-Energy Diet for Weight Loss in Overweight Adults," *International Journal of Obesity* 25, no. 10 (October 2001): 1503–11.

11 Kylie Kavanagh, DVM, et al, "Trans Fat Leads to Weight Gain Even on Same Total Calories" (presented at 66th annual Scientific Sessions of the American Diabetes Association in Washington, D.C., June 19, 2006).

12 S. P. Fowler, MPH, and colleagues at the University of Texas Health Science Center, San Antonio (data reported at the 2005 annual meeting of the American Diabetes Association in San Diego).

13 L. Wang, MD, PhD; I. Lee, MBBS, ScD; J. E. Manson, MD, DrPH; J. E. Buring, ScD; and H. D. Sesso, ScD, MPH, "Alcohol Consumption, Weight Gain, and Risk of Becoming Overweight in Middle-Aged and Older Women," *Archives of Internal Medicine* 170, no. 5 (March 2010): 453–61.

14 R. A. Breslow and B. A. Smothers, "Drinking Patterns and Body Mass Index in Never Smokers," National Health Interview Survey, 1997–2001, *American Journal of Epidemiology* 161, no. 4 (2005): 368–76.

15   A. G. Dulloo, J. Seydoux, L. Girardier, P. Chantre, and J. Vandermander, "Green Tea and Thermogenesis: Interactions between Catechin-Polyphenols, Caffeine and Sympathetic Activity," *International Journal of Obesity and Related Metabolic Disorders* 24, no. 2 (February 2000): 252–58.

16   D. Bracco, J. M. Ferrarra, M. J. Arnaud, E. Jequier, and Y. Schutz, "Effects of Caffeine on Energy Metabolism, Heart Rate, and Methylxanthine Metabolism In Lean and Obese Women," *American Journal of Physiology—Endocrinology and Metabolism* 269, no. 4 (1995): E671–E678.

17   J. Stookey, PhD, Children's Hospital and Oakland Research Institute in California (presented at the 2006 annual meeting of the Obesity Society).

18   E. R. Dove, J. M. Hodgson, I. B. Puddey, L. J. Beilin, Y. P. Lee, and T. A. Mori, "Skim Milk Compared with a Fruit Drink Acutely Reduces Appetite and Energy Intake in Overweight Men and Women," *American Journal of Clinical Nutrition* 90, no. 1 (2009): 70–75.

CHAPTER 3

1   S. M. Boback, C. L. Cox, B. D. Ott, R. Carmody, R. W. Wrangham, and S. M. Secor, "Cooking and Grinding Reduces the Cost of Meat Digestion," *Comparative Biochemistry and Physiology—Part A: Molecular & Integrative Physiology* 148, no. 3 (November 2007): 651–56.

2   K. J. Melanson, PhD, assistant professor of nutrition and food sciences at the University of Rhode Island (presented at 2007 annual meeting of the Obesity Society, New Orleans).

3   A. G. Dulloo, C. Duret, D. Rohrer, L. Girardier, N. Mensi, M. Fathi, P. Chantre, and J. Vandermander, "Efficacy of a Green Tea Extract Rich in Catechin Polyphenols and Caffeine in Increasing 24-H[our] Energy Expenditure and Fat Oxidation in Humans," *American Journal of Clinical Nutrition* 70, no. 6 (December 1999): 1040–45.

4   T. Nagao, Y. Komine, S. Soga, S. Meguro, T. Hase, Y. Tanaka, and I. Tokimitsu, "Ingestion of a Tea Rich in Catechins Leads to a Reduction in Body Fat and Malondialdehyde-Modified LDL in Men," *American Journal of Clinical Nutrition* 81, no. 1 (January 2005): 122–29.

5   D. Heber, MD, PhD, professor of medicine and public health at the UCLA Center for Human Nutrition (presented at the Experimental Biology conference April 27, 2010, Anaheim, California).

6   K. D. K. Ahuja, I. K. Robertson, D. P. Geraghty, and M. J. Ball, "Effects of Chili Consumption on Postprandial Glucose, Insulin, and Energy Metabolism," *American Journal of Clinical Nutrition* 84, no. 1 (July 2006): 63–69.

7   Judy McBride, "Cinnamon Extracts Boost Insulin Sensitivity," *Agricultural Research* (July 2000), http://www.ars.usda.gov/is/AR/archive/jul00/cinn0700.htm.

8   C. S. Johnston, I. Steplewska, C. A. Long, L. N. Harris, and R. H. Ryals, "Examination of the Antiglycemic Properties of Vinegar in Healthy Adults," *Annals of Nutrition & Metabolism* 56, no. 1 (2010): 74–79.

9   C. S. Johnston, I. Steplewska, C. A. Long, L. N. Harris, and R. H. Ryals, "Examination of the Antiglycemic Properties of Vinegar in Healthy Adults," *Annals of Nutrition and Metabolism* 56, no. 1 (2010):74–9.

CHAPTER 4

1   M. E. Bocarsly, E. S. Powell, N. M. Avena, and B. G. Hoebel, "High-Fructose Corn Syrup Causes Characteristics of Obesity in Rats: Increased Body Weight, Body Fat and Triglyceride Levels," *Pharmacology Biochemistry & Behavior* 97, no. 1 (November 2010): 101–06.

2   E. Ostman, Y. Granfeldt, L. Persson, and I. Björck, "Vinegar Supplementation Lowers Glucose and Insulin Responses and Increases Satiety after a Bread Meal in Healthy Subjects," *European Journal of Clinical Nutrition* 59 (2005): 983–88.

CHAPTER 5

1   B. Davy, PhD, associate professor of nutrition at Virginia Tech (presented at the 2010 National Meeting of the American Chemical Society in Boston).

CHAPTER 6

1   S. J. Frisbee, MSc, MA; A. Shankar, MD, PhD; S. S. Knox, PhD; K. Steenland, PhD; D. A. Savitz, PhD; T. Fletcher, PhD; A. M. Ducatman, MD, MS, "Perfluorooctanoic Acid, Perfluorooctanesulfonate, and Serum Lipids in Children and Adolescents," *Archives of Pediatrics & Adolescent Medicine* 164, no. 9 (September 2010): 860–69.

2   B. Wansink and K. van Ittersum, "The Perils of Plate Size: Waist, Waste, and Wallet," *Journal of Marketing* (2008) (under advanced review).

3   B. Wansink, K. van Ittersum, and J. E. Painter, "Ice Cream Illusions: Bowls, Spoons, and Self-Served Portion Sizes," *American Journal of Preventive Medicine* 31, no. 3 (September 2006): 240–43.

4   B. Wansink and K. van Ittersum, "Bottoms Up! The Influence of Elongation on Pouring and Consumption Volume," *Journal of Consumer Research* 30, no. 3 (December 2003): 455–63.

5   B. Wansink, "Serve Here; Eat There" (presented at 2010 Experimental Biology conference in Anaheim, California).

6   B. Wansink, J. E. Painter, and Y.-K. Lee, "The Office Candy Dish: Proximity's Influence on Estimated and Actual Consumption," *International Journal of Obesity* 30, no. 5 (May 2006): 871–75.

7   Calorie Control Council, 2000.

CHAPTER 9

1   A. H. Taylor, M. H. Ussher, and G. Faulkner, "The Acute Effects of Exercise on Cigarette Cravings, Withdrawal Symptoms, Affect and Smoking Behaviour: A Systematic Review," *Addiction* 102, no. 4 (April 2007): 534–43.

2   S. J. Elder, MS, and S. B. Roberts, PhD, "The Effects of Exercise on Food Intake and Body Fatness: A Summary of Published Studies," *Nutrition Reviews* 65, no. 1 (January 2007): 1–19.

3   D. E. Larson-Meyer, "Caloric Restriction with or without Exercise: The Fitness versus Fatness Debate," *Medicine & Science in Sports & Exercise* 42, no. 1 (January 2010): 152–59.

4   J. E. Donnelly, EdD; S. N. Blair, PED; J. M. Jakicic, PhD; M. M. Manore, PhD, RD; J. W. Rankin, PhD; and B. K. Smith, PhD, "Appropriate Physical Activity Intervention Strategies for Weight Loss and Prevention of Weight Regain for Adults," *Medicine & Science in Sports & Exercise* 41, no. 2 (February 2009): 459–71.

5   L. M. Fenicchia, J. A. Kanaley, J. L. Azevedo Jr, C. S. Miller, R. S. Weinstock, R. L. Carhart, and L. L. Ploutz-Snyder, "Influence of Resistance Exercise Training on Glucose Control in Women with Type 2 Diabetes," *Metabolism,* 53, no. 3 (March 2004): 284–89.

6   W. K. Mummery, PhD; G. M. Schofield, PhD; R. Steele, BHSc; E. G. Eakin, PhD; and W. J. Brown, PhD, "Occupational Sitting Time and Overweight and Obesity in Australian Workers," *American Journal of Preventive Medicine* 29, no. 2 (August 2005): 91–97.

7   R. W. Boyce, E. L. Boone, B. W. Cioci, and A. H. Lee, "Physical Activity, Weight Gain and Occupational Health among Call Centre Employees," *Occupational Medicine* 58, no. 4 (2008): 238–44.

8   T. Y. Warren, V. Barry, S. P. Hooker, X. Sui, T. S. Church, and S. N. Blair, "Sedentary Behaviors Increase Risk of Cardiovascular Disease Mortality in Men," *Medicine & Science in Sports & Exercise* 42, no. 5 (May 2010): 879–85.

9   J. A. Levine, L. M. Lanningham-Foster, S. K. McCrady, A C. Krizan, L. R. Olson, P. H. Kane, M. D. Jensen, and M. M. Clark, "Interindividual Variation in Posture Allocation: Possible Role in Human Obesity," *Science* 307, no. 5709 (January 28, 2005): 584–86.

10 B. Braun, PhD, associate professor in the department of kinesiology, University of Massachusetts–Amherst (unpublished).

11 F. B. Hu, MD, PhD; T. Y. Li, MD; G. A. Colditz, MD, DrPH; W. C. Willett, MD, DrPH; and J. E. Manson, MD, DrPH, "Television Watching and Other Sedentary Behaviors in Relation to Risk of Obesity and Type 2 Diabetes Mellitus in Women," *Journal of the American Medical Association* 289, no. 14 (April 9, 2003): 1785–91.

12 R. E. Andersen, PhD; S. C. Franckowiak, BS; J. Snyder, BS; S. J. Bartlett, PhD; and K. R. Fontaine, PhD, "Can Inexpensive Signs Encourage the Use of Stairs?" *Annals of Internal Medicine* 129, no. 5 (September 1, 1998): 363–69.

13 Interview with Joyce A. Hanna, associate director of the Health Improvement Program at Stanford University, Palo Alto, California, 4/16/99.

14 A. L. Dunn, PhD; B. H. Marcus, PhD; J. B. Kampert, PhD; M. E. Garcia, MPH; H. W. Kohl III, PhD; and S. N. Blair, PED, "Comparison of Lifestyle and Structured Interventions to Increase Physical Activity and Cardiorespiratory Fitness," *Journal of the American Medical Association* 281, no. 4 (January 27, 1999): 327–34.

15 D. A. McAlpine, C. U. Manohar, S. K. McCrady, D. Hensrud, and J. A. Levine, "An Office-Place Stepping Device to Promote Workplace Physical Activity," *British Journal of Sports Medicine* 41, no. 12 (December 2007): 903–7.

CHAPTER 10

1   H. Wyatt, MD, an endocrinology professor at the University of Colorado, Denver, presented to the 2002 National Association for the Study of Obesity.

2   D. Berry, PhD, RN, "Women Maintaining Weight Loss," *Nursing Science Quarterly* 17, no. 3 (July 2004): 242–52.

3   S. Kayman, W. Bruvold, and J. S. Stern, "Maintenance and Relapse after Weight Loss in Women: Behavioral Aspects," *American Journal of Clinical Nutrition* 52, no. 5 (November 1990): 800–7.

Index

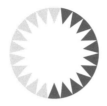

Underscored page references indicate boxed text and tables.
Boldface references indicate photographs and illustrations.

INDEX

Fullness. *See also* Satiety
    from carbonated water, 40
    ranking, 248

G

Garlic
    Honey-Glazed Pork Loin with Garlic Mashed
        Potatoes, 169
    lemon garlic chicken thighs with tarragon,
        327
    as warming food, 43
Garlic press, 89
Ginger
    Carrot-Ginger Soup with Cashews and
        Chicken, 125
    cinnamon-ginger oatmeal, 304
    as warming food, 43
Ginger peeler, 89
Glasses, downsizing, 91
Good Grips Salad Chopper and Bowl, 87
Grace before meals, 94
Grains. *See* Whole grains
Grazing, problems with, 9–10
Green tea, 31–32, 40–41
Griffin, Deborah, 206–7, **206**, **207**
Grill basket, 87
Grilling foods, 87
Grocery shopping, 62–63, 65, 66–67, 83
Guilt, about eating, 13
Gum chewing, for weight loss, 37

H

Ham
    Cuban Sandwich, 137
    Ham-and-Cheese Bake, 116
    ham and cheese sandwich, 318
Hearty foods, Active Calories in, 4, 36, 37, 40
HFCS. *See* High fructose corn syrup
High-fiber foods, as Active Calories, xiv–xv
High fructose corn syrup (HFCS), 51, 61, 84
Honey
    Honey-Glazed Pork Loin with Garlic Mashed
        Potatoes, 169
Household chores, as exercise, 242
Hummus
    Black Bean Hummus with Toasted Pita, 180
Hunger
    breakfast preventing, 9
    exercise reducing, 216
    fat preventing, 25
    minimeals interfering with, 10
    resistant starches and, 22

Hunger scale, 90, 247–48
    in Active Calorie Diet Journal, 264–65

I

Ice cream
    Easy Ice Cream Sandwiches, 191
Insulin, 42, 46, 48, 54, 55

J

Jalapeño chile peppers
    Corn Muffins with Colby and Jalapeño, 182
Jerky, 18
Johnson, Jeannette, 88–89
Journaling. *See also* Active Calorie Diet Journal
    purpose of, xvii–xviii, 98–99, 246, 263
Juices, fruit, xv, 47

K

Kebabs
    beef and vegetable kebabs, 317
KFC, Active Calorie choices at, 197–98
Kitchen
    de-cluttering, 98
    food storage in, 95–97
Kitchen tools, 83, 84, 85–86, 87–88, 89–90
Knives, 83, 84

L

Labels, food, reading, 84
Lighting, during meals, 97–98
Linguine
    Shrimp Scampi Linguine, 174
Liquid calories, 30–33
Lunch, 122–23
    additions to, for men, 64
    Avocado Seafood Salad, 132
    Barbecue Chicken Salad, 131
    best fast food, 195, 196, 197, 198, 199, 200,
        201, 202, 203, 204
    Black Bean Burger, 139
    California Salad, 128
    calories from, 60
    Carrot-Ginger Soup with Cashews and
        Chicken, 125
    Chicken Minestrone, 124
    Chili-Topped Sweet Potato, 145
    Cuban Sandwich, 137
    Egg Salad, 127
    Mini Meatball Soup, 126
    Miso Beef and Noodles, 149

It's Not About Counting Calories
It's About Making Them Count!

The Active Calorie Diet™ is the revolutionary new 4-week program from *Prevention* that lets you eat more, burn more, and lose more WITHOUT counting calories, all while eating REAL food! Firmly grounded in science, the Active Calorie Diet helps you drop one dress size or more!

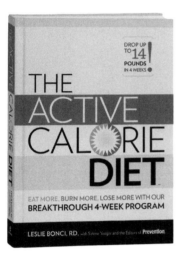

- **DISCOVER THE SECRET** to activating your calories and losing big!

- **GET MORE ENERGY** from your food with the CHEW factor!

- **DISCOVER DELICIOUS RECIPES** and smart on-the-go eats!

- **LOSE MORE** with effective strength-training, stretching, and cardio exercises

- **AND MUCH MORE!**

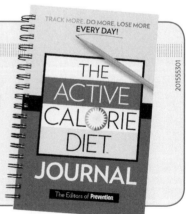

ALSO AVAILABLE:

The Active Calorie Diet™ *Journal*
Make every calorie count without counting calories! Intensify your Active Calorie Diet results by recording your results, what you're eating, and your exercises in this comprehensive journal!

Visit www.prevention.com/shop or call *Prevention* Customer Service at (800) 848-4735 to order your copies today!